OFFICE CALLS

•And Other Stories From Thirty
Years of Rural Medicine •

Gary Yarbrough, M.D.
- author of "House Calls" -

Dedication

This book is dedicated to Dianne, my nurse and my spouse.

Forward

After the warm reception of my first book, "House Calls", many friends and readers implored me to write more stories about medical cases I have known. That first book was given excellent reviews on Amazon, the most common complaint being, "It was too short!" In a way that was a compliment, indicating to me that the stories were enjoyed, but the reader wanted more of them.

Frankly, making house calls has not consumed the major part of my time in medicine. Although some of the stories in this second book take place in a hospital setting, most of my work as a physician has taken place in the office, thus the title "Office Calls - and other stories". With the writing of this book I have been able to share with you, the reader, those things that happen in the settings where most family doctors spend most of their professional lives.

Once again, I have changed names and circumstances to try to protect the privacy of the persons whose stories you are about to read. It is my hope that no one will recognize themselves or those they know in reading them, but that everyone will enjoy reading them.

Gary Yarbrough, M.D.
Parsons, Kansas
October 2013

Table Of Contents

Table Of Contents (Continued)

Adhesions

Eugene Wertzler was a broken, bitter, angry man, verbally and physically abusive to his wife, Anna, and their son Roger. He wasn't always that way, according to Anna. They had married when she was sixteen and he was twenty-one and employed at a local factory. As Anna was pregnant at the time, they decided to elope to keep their parents from finding out about it. During their first several months together, all seemed to be going well for them, until their son was born with a club foot and mild mental retardation. Eugene always looked upon Roger as his punishment from God for Anna's having been pregnant before their marriage. Sadly, Eugene and Anna were never able to have more children.

When Roger was just three years old and undergoing his second operation on his club foot, the factory union to which Eugene belonged went on strike. Unfortunately, Eugene felt he could not do without his regular wages to make ends meet. He decided to cross the picket line to work his regular evening shift. Two weeks later, while the strike was still on, he was brutally beaten by a group of union men wielding baseball bats.

Severely injured with multiple fractures, he was hospitalized for several weeks after the incident. He never fully regained the use of his left leg or right arm. He could not fully straighten his left leg and had to walk tiptoe on the left with a bad limp. He was unable to return to regular work, leaving him bitter and angry at life, an anger he took out on those closest to him, Anna and Roger. Sadly, the men who had beaten him so badly were never identified or brought to justice.

With her husband no longer able to work, Anna, who was working as an aide at a nursing home, began attending evening classes to complete her training to become a licensed practical nurse, or LPN. Once she finished and was licensed, she worked in that capacity for several nursing homes. Her income and Eugene's modest disability check were just enough to keep the family together. I learned all of this history when Anna first came to see me several years ago at age sixty for right upper abdominal pain. An ultrasound revealed she had gallstones and thickening of the gallbladder wall. I referred her to a local surgeon who removed the diseased organ, and she seemed to recover without problem. However, about six months later, she returned due to abnormal uterine bleeding. The gynecologist to whom I referred her found that Anna had pre-cancerous tissue and needed a hysterectomy. Unfortunately, at that operation Anna was found to have widespread dense adhesions, all of which had to be released carefully before the hysterectomy could even be started.

Postoperative abdominal adhesions are a very common cause of pain and bowel obstruction. These adhesions are scar tissues between bowel loops, onto the lining of the abdominal wall (the peritoneum), or with other organs within the abdominal cavity, as was the case for Anna. They are believed to be caused by inflammation on the surface of the abdominal organs due to handling at the time of surgery, a foreign object inside the abdomen, bleeding into the abdominal cavity, or certain gynecologic conditions such as pelvic inflammatory disease or endometriosis. Normally the loops of the intestines move around freely within the abdomen, sliding over each other and over surrounding organs on a thin film of fluid. Once adhesions have formed, the bowel loops are no longer able to move freely and may become twisted or trapped. An intestine entrapped or twisted upon itself causes significant pain and, if severe enough, partial or complete obstruction of the small bowel.

Most of the time bowel obstruction due to adhesions is intermittent and often can reverse itself spontaneously. Sometimes the obstruction resolves with eating or by passing stool or gas. When it persists, the patient typically develops a colicky discomfort around the umbilicus, or belly button, with gradually worsening pain and eventually distention of the abdomen. This leads to nausea and vomiting. Anna had not known she had adhesions until after her hysterectomy. She then recalled how she often had had vague abdominal pain and bloating since the gallbladder surgery, which she had attributed to the absence of gallbladder. Unfortunately, this was just the beginning of Anna's trouble from adhesions.

About four years after her hysterectomy Anna developed left lower abdominal pain with fever and bowel obstruction. She underwent emergency surgery with removal of a foot of her colon due to the rupture of a diverticular abscess. Rupture of the colon like this is the worst complication of diverticulosis. Once again, the surgeon found dense adhesions throughout Anna's abdomen, locking down multiple loops of small intestine over the area of the ruptured colon. All these bowel loops had to be freed up carefully to access the ruptured colon. Her hospital stay was prolonged and stormy due to the spillage of stool into the abdominal cavity from the ruptured colon, but she eventually recovered and resumed working.

After that episode, almost once a year Anna had to be admitted to the hospital for mechanical bowel obstruction (also called mechanical ileus) due to adhesions. Fortunately, during most of these admissions, the obstruction could be relieved with the placement of a nasogastric tube through her nose and into her stomach to deflate the bowel and put it to rest, along with intravenous fluids to keep her hydrated. However, occasionally these measures were not sufficient to relieve the problem. In those instances, to avoid another open abdominal surgery, she had to have a Gastrografin small bowel x-ray series.

Gastrografin is the brand name of a water soluble x-ray contrast liquid that contains a large amount organic iodine. Since iodine has a very high atomic weight, it produces enough density to x-rays to give a white shadow contrasting with the surrounding tissues. Because of its high iodine content, Gastrografin has to be used with caution in patients with thyroid disease. In addition Gastrograffin is hypertonic, or concentrated, compared to plasma. As a result, it causes brisk diffusion of water into the lumen or opening of the bowel. This acts like an osmotic laxative, leading to considerable pressure within the bowel to relieve the obstruction, followed by a torrential diarrhea.

The Gastrografin small bowel x-ray series was very effective in relieving Anna's bowel obstruction. Three times she developed obstruction that would not relieve itself with a nasogastric tube and bowel rest. Each time the contrast medium would finally pass through the twisted intestine, causing an explosive diarrhea, stopping her pain and relieving her distention. Anna wasn't particularly happy about the watery diarrhea, but she was relieved that she didn't require another surgery. Indeed, she had once told me she would never again agree to surgery, having had so much trouble with adhesions from her previous ones.

Unfortunately, the fourth time she was given Gastrografin, it failed to relieve her obstruction. Her pain continued to worsen until she finally agreed to surgery, since her only other option at that point was hospice care. Moreover, Eugene had died earlier that year from a massive stroke, so she was the only one left to take care of Roger. In the operating room she was found to have a perforated loop of small bowel due to severe dilation from the obstruction. Fortunately, she recovered from that operation without much difficulty. Anna is now retired from nursing home work. In addition to her Social Security check Roger brings home a small income from his work as a dishwasher, and they seem to be happier with Eugene gone. Anna continues to have episodes of partial bowel obstruction almost annually, but so far the Gastrografin has prevented her from needing another surgery.

Even as of this writing there is still no treatment proven to prevent diffuse abdominal adhesions after surgery. Adhesions tend to recur, especially for patients like Anna who have a strong tendency to form them. The very process of releasing the loops of bowel is believed to cause new inflammation and the formation of new adhesions. A product called Seprafilm is now used to prevent abdominal organs from sticking to the incision line inside on the peritoneum, but there is still no way to prevent widespread adhesions deeper in the abdomen. Perhaps someday a product will be developed to prevent these adhesions for patients like Anna.

Anaphylaxis

One of the most exciting office cases I've ever had was brought to us courtesy of an unfriendly bumblebee that stung a twenty-eight year-old fellow named Stanley.

Stanley and his friend were fishing along the Ohio River when the bumblebee landed on Stan's neck and stung him. This bumblebee attack was witnessed by his friend. Unfortunately, Stan had a history of bad reactions to bee stings and started having his worst reaction ever with this bumblebee's sting.

His friend helped him into his pickup truck and drove him the six miles from their fishing spot on the river to town. He initially took Stan to another medical office in town, but there he was refused treatment. Unfortunately, Stan was a very irresponsible young man and had never even made payments on his bills at that office. They had sent him a letter telling him to find another doctor and that they would no longer see him. His friend then drove him the three blocks to my office and helped him in the door.

Stan was a tall stout man with sandy-blond hair, an unshaven sandy-brown beard (back before the unkempt look was popular), and sunburned face. He was shaking, soaked with sweat, and spoke with very slurred speech as his face, neck, and tongue were already swollen from the bumblebee sting. His eyes were narrow slits from the swelling, so it was hard for him to see where he was walking. By then he was so lightheaded that he could just barely tell us his name and that he had been stung by the bumblebee.

My medical assistant obtained the remainder of his information, such as his address, telephone number, and the like, from his friend while the nurse and I assisted Stan down the short hallway to the treatment room. We managed to get him stumbling and shuffling to the room, but we practically had to lift him onto the treatment table as he was losing consciousness. His breathing became extremely labored, rapid, and so shallow that the nurse thought he had stopped breathing. Stan was, of course, suffering from acute anaphylactic shock.

Anaphylactic shock is the most severe form of allergic reaction. Approximately 2,000 people die each year in this country from systemic anaphylaxis. Nonfatal cases are much more common. Anaphylaxis can occur in response to any number of allergens. It is more likely to happen with injected allergens than with an allergen, like a pollen, landing on a mucous membrane, though it can occur with ingested allergens, particularly in children (and some adults) with food allergies. Anaphylaxis never occurs unless the patient has been exposed to the allergen repeatedly prior to having the anaphylactic response. The Hymenoptera family of bees, hornets, wasps, and fire ants are much more likely than other allergens to produce anaphylactic reactions such as Stan experienced.

There are in the body certain cells, known as mast cells, which contain histamine granules and other chemicals of severe allergy. When an individual has been sensitized to an allergen by repeated exposure in the past, the mast cells will be coated with immune antibody or IgE. This is the immunoprotein in the blood created in reaction to an allergen.

When the venom is injected into the body, it interacts with the IgE on the mast cells, causing massive release of histamine and other allergic chemicals. These chemicals then react with receptors on the cells lining blood vessels, smooth muscle cells, and nerve cells. This then produces bronchial constriction, wheezing, and shortness of breath, gastrointestinal cramping, and increased blood vessel permeability. All of these are associated with oozing of fluid from tissue cells, causing the initial massive swelling such as Stan had on his face and neck, and loss of fluid from the blood circulation leading to a dramatic drop in blood pressure.

There is also intense itching, or pruritus, with various red rashes and hives, known as urticaria. Because of the effects on digestive organs, the patient may also have nausea, vomiting, and diarrhea. The massive sweating, called diaphoresis, also results in further fluid loss and contributes to the extremely low blood pressure and shock. In Stan's case his initial blood pressure was 50/0 when we finally had him lying down on the treatment table. Clearly he was in danger of imminent death if we did not institute resuscitation treatment at once. Any more delay and Stan would have left the office in one of the funeral director's bags.

I told my nurse to prepare a liter bag of normal saline while I reached for our emergency drugs. The first thing I did was to inject Stan in one of his thighs with epinephrine. I then connected him to oxygen and opened the oxygen bottle to the fastest flow rate we could give him. I next injected Stan's other thigh with benadryl, a potent antihistamine, to slow down the allergic reaction. By that time the nurse had started his IV, which we ran wide open as fast as it would infuse. I was now able to give Stan a second dose of epinephrine through the IV line.

Other than the infusion of fluids as fast as possible to support circulation, epinephrine, also called adrenaline, is the most important medication in anaphylaxis. The earlier it is given the better. There are even epinephrine pens that those with severe allergies can carry with them to prevent anaphylactic shock. The benadryl, an antihistamine, would not begin working immediately like epinephrine, but the sooner we gave it, the sooner it would help. Finally, I gave Stan Solu Medrol through his IV and an injection of Depo Medrol in his buttock. These steroid medications would also not work immediately; however, the sooner they were given, the sooner they would begin helping.

Within minutes of getting his second shot of epinephrine, Stanley began breathing better and started to arouse. His blood pressure began rising as well. We breathed sighs of relief, as the nurse and I realized Stan had gotten to us just in the nick of time. After he began breathing better, I had the nurse give Stan a nebulizer treatment with albuterol, a bronchodilator, and this further improved him to where he was breathing comfortably.

After the infusion of a full liter of IV fluid, Stan was feeling much better. He was breathing normally. His blood pressure was back up to 100/60. I recommended to Stan that he go by ambulance to the hospital, twenty-six miles away, but he refused. He said he couldn't afford it. He told me he was living on welfare but did not have Medicaid.

I advised him he was really not out of the woods yet from this anaphylactic reaction, but he insisted he would be fine. He refused any other treatment except for a prescription for corticosteroid tablets and benadryl, which at that time was not available over-the-counter. He signed a form refusing further care and left in the company of his friend.

Ironically, though he had been in danger of sudden death and was one of the sickest patients we have ever treated, he never paid his bill, which, back then, was just under a hundred dollars, for all we had done for him.

It still amazes me that someone could feel that their life wasn't worth a hundred dollars. Perhaps even more amazing was the refusal of the other medical office in town to treat a man on the verge of death simply because he had not paid his old bill.

Anointing

Upon moving to Parsons, Kansas my wife and I became parishioners at St. Patrick's Catholic Church. At first there was an older priest here as pastor, but within a few years he was transferred by the Bishop. A new young priest, Father Smith, was assigned to us as pastor. This was only his second assignment since ordination and his first as a pastor. He was in a new role, in a new town, meeting new people for the first time. To get to know the people of his new parish he made it a point to visit at each parishioner's home during his first year at St. Patrick's. Father Smith was seen right away to be a very holy man, with a deep prayer life and a great reverence for the sacraments. Though he took very seriously his role as pastor, he had a great sense of humor as well.

Dianne and I enjoyed his visit to our house, and Father apparently did as well. He seemed impressed that all was tidy, and asked Dianne if she had ever done work as a sacristan in the past. The sacristan is the person who maintains the sacred vessels and the linens used at Mass. He was not happy with the prior custom of using the same linens for a whole week and wanted to find someone to take care of things so that he would have a clean set of linens for each Mass. Dianne had done some work for a short time years before for her uncle who was a priest. She agreed to take on the task. She bought a book that taught her how to do the job, and from the outset Father Smith was very pleased with her work. I also helped out with polishing the sacred vessels, candle lighters, and thuribles, and both of us quickly became good friends with the new young priest. We would often joke and tease one another back and forth.

Back then we still had not obtained full-time emergency room doctors, so, along with the other family physicians in town, I would take my turn on call for the emergency room in rotation. One day when it was my turn on call, after finishing work at the office I went to the emergency room and stayed seeing patients until everyone had been taken care of. Finally, at 10:30 that night we had no more patients, and I went on home. The nurse assured me she would call right away should a patient come in for treatment.

The phone on the bedside table rang at 1:30 that morning. It was the ER nurse. She had just received a radio call from an ambulance crew on its way from Columbus, Kansas, with an elderly lady in full cardiac arrest. A long-time cardiac patient, she had been having chest pain that evening and finally could not stop it with nitroglycerin. Living alone, she had called the ambulance herself but went into complete arrest shortly after they arrived at her home. The EMTs had started an IV, begun CPR, and were bagging her. They would arrive shortly. I quickly dressed, hurried down stairs, and drove as prudently but quickly as possible to the hospital. I was pleased to have arrived there before the ambulance.

The experienced emergency room nurse had already assembled the laboratory technician, respiratory therapy technician, and the nursing supervisor. It was she who would obtain medications from the hospital pharmacy should we need them. I quickly reviewed with the staff all the protocols for Advanced Cardiac Life Support, known as ACLS. Though all of us present had been trained in ACLS, I felt it didn't hurt to review the standard protocols prior to the arrival of our patient. It might have been a few years since some of the staff had last been recertified, and the review might be appreciated.

Not long after I arrived the ambulance crew drove up to the entrance with the patient in "full code". We wheeled her into our cardiac room while the EMTs continued CPR. The nurse quickly hooked her to our electronic monitor and found she was in ventricular fibrillation, a life-threatening pulseless rhythm. I quickly prepared the defibrillator, called, "All clear!" and shocked her heart; she remained in ventricular fibrillation. This process was repeated two more times. Each time the defibrillation was unsuccessful. Her heart continued to fibrillate. Though the ambulance crew was doing a good job of breathing for her with the ventilating bag, I inserted an endotracheal tube. This tube, passing through the mouth and into the windpipe, can not only be used for breathing for her but would also protect her airway from stomach contents getting into the lungs during the resuscitation efforts.

We started a second IV line in addition to the one started by the ambulance crew and, following the ACLS protocols, tried several intravenous heart medications, each medication followed by CPR to circulate it and then another electric shock to the patient's heart. As we continued following our way through the ACLS protocols, it became clear we were not making progress. Sadly, though we did finally get our patient's rhythm to change, it was into the rhythm of a dying heart. This rhythm is basically a flatline tracing with only occasional electrical activity which does not result in contraction of the heart muscle. It was apparent there was nothing more that could be done. By now it was three in the morning.

I asked the respiratory therapist to continue bagging her while we went through her purse to see if we could find any next of kin. We did not find information on her next of kin but did find holy cards and her rosary, indicating that our patient was a Catholic. I immediately called the rectory at St. Patrick's, waking up Father Smith, and advising him that we needed him at the ER to anoint a dying patient. Knowing how we had teased one another in the past, Father said, "Doc, is this your idea of a joke?" I informed him it was no joke; we were awaiting his arrival to the ER as soon as he could come.

Something in my voice must have convinced him this was real, for it did not take him long to arrive. As Father came through the doors, I instructed the respiratory therapist to stop bagging the patient. We extubated her (removed the endotracheal tube from her throat) and made her more presentable but left her connected to the monitor. We closed the door part way to give them some privacy.

We were all sitting at the nursing station writing up everything that we had done, documenting the "code blue" cardiac arrest treatment process as best we could. Such times are always of high stress, and we all appreciated the chronological record the nursing supervisor had recorded. Suddenly we all about jumped out of our seats. As the priest was anointing her, our patient's heart suddenly began beating again on its own! We heard her cardiac monitor suddenly start beeping, initially at a slow rate, then speeding up to normal!

We rushed into the room and found not only did our patient have a spontaneous heartbeat, but she also had a pulse with it and had begun breathing on her own! Father looked up at me in surprise, almost as if to say, "I thought you said she was dying!" I informed him that she indeed was dying; we had done all we could to resuscitate her, using the best available protocols for treatment, with no success. Yet as he began anointing her, her heart had resumed beating on its own. As I spoke with him, she gradually regained consciousness, started speaking to us, and asked us where she was and what had happened. To my surprise she even complained that she had not been taken to another nearby hospital where her doctor practiced. We were happy to contact her doctor and transfer her to that hospital, now that she was stable and alert.

For several years this lady exchanged Christmas cards with Father Smith. He told me that he finally stopped getting cards from her. We both suspected she may have finally died, and both of us assumed it would have been from heart disease. That night in the emergency room was surely a lesson to me about the limits of what medicine can do and the power of sacramental prayers.

Arachnoiditis

Bert had called with complaint of severe low back pain shooting like electric shocks down the backs of his legs since lifting a deer from his hunting trip the evening before. That morning he awoke barely able to walk. The nurse asked Bert to come for an appointment at one o'clock that afternoon, working him into our schedule. When he arrived, he moved very slowly, bent forward at the waist, obviously in great pain, in spite of which he managed to joke that he now had a new occupation as a "carpet inspector". The nurse helped him into the exam room and onto a table. On examination I found he had weakness in raising up his right foot. His "electric shock" pains were in the distribution of the L4, L5 and S1 nerve roots. This was true sciatica for which he would need an MRI of his lumbar spine. I wrote him the first of what would become many prescriptions for pain medication, and we scheduled his MRI.

Bert was a tall lanky gentleman I had first met through church organizations. A Vietnam veteran, he had run a local financial institution but was now retired due to post-traumatic stress disorder. However, he still remained active with hunting, fishing, and a sideline taxidermy business. He was a strong man with a steady penetrating gaze, thinning light brown hair, and a winning smile. Other men I had met through church told me Bert was one of the best shots they had ever seen on bird hunts. He could also sharpen a blade better than anyone. Unfortunately, now he could do none of those activities due to the great pain he was suffering. We were able to get his MRI scheduled for the next day; it showed two bulging spinal discs and two more massively herniated with extruded material pressing against multiple nerve roots.

A spinal disc is built much like a jelly doughnut. The outer casing, the annulus fibrosis, is a very tough springy material with little stretch to it. The "jelly" inside, nucleus pulposus, has the consistency of old jello that has been left in the refrigerator a few weeks. This firm rubbery material provides the shock absorbing cushioning between vertebrae when we jump down from a height. Now the nucleus pulposus of two of them had been squeezed out and was pressing hard against nerve roots while the annulus fibrosis of another two were bulging into nerve roots, all of which contributed to the pain down his legs. Because of the extensive nature of his back damage, surgery was Bert's best option. I referred him to a neurosurgeon for evaluation and treatment. After being seen by the neurosurgeon, Bert was scheduled for surgery with spinal fusion at four different levels. We expected him to do well.

Unfortunately, Bert had pain relief for just a couple of days. His pain returned with a vengeance and in addition to the electric shock-like shooting pains down the legs, he developed tingling, weakness, and numbness with muscle spasms and at times uncontrollable twitching. He also found it much more difficult to empty his bladder. Bert soon began requiring more and more pain pills to control his symptoms. I knew him well and knew he was not an addict or drug seeker, so I wrote him prescriptions for enough pain medication to keep him as functional as possible. Bert returned to the neurosurgeon for his follow-up visit and was immediately sent for another MRI. Unfortunately, this confirmed the diagnosis suspected by the neurosurgeon, chronic adhesive arachnoiditis.

Chronic adhesive arachnoiditis is a disorder of extreme pain caused by inflammation of the arachnoid, one of the three meninges, or membranes, surrounding the brain and spinal cord. The pia mater is the most internal layer. It covers the surface of the brain and spinal cord, so closely adherent that it cannot be dissected from them. Next is the subarachnoid space filled with cerebrospinal fluid, and above this is the arachnoid membrane. It is a delicate transparent membrane with small branches, or trabeculations, connecting it with the pia mater. Outside the arachnoid is the dura mater, a thick dense fibrous layer enclosing and protecting all the rest. For reasons still unknown, after spinal surgery some patients develop inflammation and adhesions of the arachnoid that compress the spinal cord and nerve roots. This scarring causes the severe intractable pain of adhesive arachnoiditis. In a sense this is comparable to the formation of peritoneal adhesions seen after abdominal surgery.

Diagnosing arachnoiditis can be difficult but the second MRI had confirmed Bert's diagnosis. Additional testing such as with an EMG/NCS, or electromyogram/nerve conduction study, can assess the severity of the ongoing damage to the affected nerve roots. Often there is little reason to perform such additional testing since there is no cure for arachnoiditis and the only treatment is pain management.

Treatment options for arachnoiditis are identical to those for other chronic pain conditions. Any surgery for arachnoiditis is controversial, because the outcome is often very poor and provides only short-term relief. Initially Bert was tried with a TENS unit, Transcutaneous Electrical Nerve Stimulator, but it was ineffective. We then tried Bert on a variety of medications, including low-dose tricyclic antidepressants. These are used in doses inadequate to relieve depression, but enough to change the way the brain perceives pain. For those with chronic nerve pain this can provide significant relief. Such patients will say, " I hurt just as bad on the medication, but it doesn't bother me much now." Interestingly, the old tricyclic antidepressants are dramatically more effective than the newer types of antidepressants, such as Prozac; these do not work well. Other medications we tried with Bert included anti-seizure medications, as these can also affect away the brain perceives pain and provide some patients with substantial relief. However, we tried two different ones with Bert, and neither one helped. Low-dose benzodiazepine medications, such as Valium or Xanax, can be used when muscle spasms are prominent, but Bert did not need them very often.

Unfortunately, Bert called me this last year with complaint of urinating air. He apparently had developed a diverticular abscess which formed a fistula, or abnormal connection, between his colon and bladder. As he was taking the pain medication for his back, Bert did not feel the pain normally associated with this. He had to undergo surgery twice, once to remove the affected section of colon and close the fistula, along with having a temporary colostomy; the second surgery reversed the colostomy. Fortunately, he has done well since then.

I continue to adjust Bert's pain medication and as much as possible to try to control his symptoms without causing excessive sedation or side effects, but he still has significant trouble with constipation with any dosage. He has had to use chronic laxatives to deal with that. In addition, three years ago Bert sought relief by having a spinal stimulator implanted, but this proved to be completely ineffective. He finally had it removed last year.

We now have Bert fairly well regulated on long-acting morphine every 12 hours with short acting oxycodone in between for breakthrough pain. He still has to use chronic laxatives, and he is still at risk for complications from the chronic use of narcotics. However, it at least keeps his pain fairly well in check so that he is able to do some work around the house. He still walks bent over at the waist and calls himself a carpet inspector. If he is on his feet very long, his pain is significantly worse. Sadly, there is nothing

else that I can do for him. His is one of the saddest cases I
have seen in thirty years as a doctor.

Asthma

In the mid 1980s the University of Florida put on an intensive annual Family Medicine Review each year in Orlando, Florida. The program, always held at a large hotel near the Disney World complex, offered up to fifty hours of continuing medical education, or CME. This met the requirements of almost all state licensing boards for CME. Thus a physician could meet the CME requirement for a whole year in just a few days and enjoy a visit or two to Disney World as well.

In 1987 I attended this program with Dianne, my wife and office nurse. We had managed to arrange sitters for our children so we could take the trip alone together. We flew to Orlando, prepared to spend long hours in the lecture hall, but looking forward to afternoons and evenings at Disney World. Years prior, before we were married, we often went on dates to Disneyland in Anaheim, California. Now we would have our first opportunity to experience Walt Disney's other theme park while I met my CME requirements for the state of Michigan at the same time.

The first few days there were very busy with lectures on a wide variety of medical topics. On the third day we had a late afternoon and evening open to ourselves. We took this opportunity to make our first foray into Disney World. Fortunately, our hotel ran a shuttle bus to the park several times a day, including one that would run late at night as the park was closing. Having eaten hotel food the last few days, we decided we would eat supper at Disney World. We found the food there was wonderful. After our meal we spent several enjoyable hours touring the many exhibits, watching several live shows, and shopping in the many international shops. Of course, we also had to purchase several Disney-related items for our children back home. As it was getting late, we decided to wait to see the famous fireworks show the park put on each night. We stood by the lake and got to see it twice, once in the sky and again in the reflection from the calm lake water! The display was truly beautiful. Afterward the park would be closing, so we made our way back to the main gate to await our hotel shuttle bus.

By the time we arrived at the front gate, our shuttle bus was already filled, mostly with other doctors and their families. The driver said he would make another run back since there were so many from the hotel that had gone to Disney World that evening. We didn't mind waiting to be in the second load. The evening was soft with a wispy ground fog slowly drifting out from over the lake into the parking area. We were enjoying the chance to talk over all the things we had seen in Disney World and at the Epcot Center.

As we stood there talking and awaiting the return of the hotel bus, Dianne noticed about twenty yards to our right a young girl apparently having trouble breathing. She was standing on the sidewalk with her mother and younger brother, the three of them also apparently waiting for a shuttle bus from a different hotel. When Dianne pointed out this girl to me, we both walked down the sidewalk to where they were standing. We introduced ourselves, and informed the mother, Mrs. Patterson, that I was a doctor and Dianne a nurse. Both of the Patterson children, Frances age 13 and Thomas age nine, suffered from asthma. They had traveled from Wisconsin to Orlando for the Disney trip without Mr. Patterson, who could not get away from work. Frances had left her inhaler at their hotel but had tried using her brother's; however, it was not helping. I ran back to the main gate where the park attendant had just finished locking it. I explained to him how Frances urgently needed first aid assistance, but his reply was, "I'm sorry. The park is closed." To this day I am dismayed that a theme park bearing the name of Walt Disney would be so family unfriendly.

I went back to where our group was standing and advised Mrs. Patterson we needed to hail a cab to take her daughter to the nearest urgent care center. I managed to get the attention of a cab driver, but he spoke mostly Cuban. Having studied collegiate Spanish, however, I was able to remember enough to explain to him we needed to go to the nearest urgent care center right away. Mrs. Patterson was reluctant to go at first, as she wasn't sure she had enough money for the cab fare. Dianne and I offered to help pay for it, so she accepted, and we all took off in the one cab.

We were quickly driven from Disney World through the streets of Orlando, and within a few minutes we were at an urgent care center. Unfortunately, just a few minutes before we had arrived, the urgent care center had also closed.

Sitting in the cab in front of the closed urgent care center, little Frances was getting progressively worse. In addition, now her younger brother, Thomas, started having problems with his asthma as he was frightened for his sister. Dianne noticed that, in his anxiety, he was using his own inhaler to excess. Dianne asked Thomas what prayers he knew, and he mentioned Catholic prayers familiar to all of us. Dianne had him start reciting these prayers to ask God to help his sister, and this seemed to calm him down. Saying those prayers gave him something helpful to do in this stressful situation.

Hearing Frances trying to breathe, the cab driver understood when I told him we needed to get to a hospital now; he began driving again. Frances was getting worse with each passing minute. It was when I noticed she was turning a little blue, barely moving air and looking semi-conscious, that I yelled at the cab driver to stop at once. He pulled to the curb in front of a motel. As I laid Frances out on their cool wet grass, I had Dianne run to the night window. She had the attendant call 911, to tell them where we were, and that we had a little girl with an asthma attack going unconscious. I began to give Frances mouth-to-mouth breathing, blowing air as best I could through her tight airways. Fortunately, in less than five minutes the ambulance arrived. I immediately advised the EMTs of Frances' diagnosis of "status asthmaticus", the worst stage of asthma. She need an adrenaline shot right away. The EMT advised me he needed a doctor's order for that. Thankfully, when I identified myself as a physician visiting from Michigan, he agreed to give her the epinephrine injection, and at the dosage I had recommended. She was started on oxygen, loaded onto their cart, and lifted into the ambulance. Fortunately the EMTs also agreed to transport Mrs. Patterson and Thomas to the children's hospital, just six blocks away. The night attendant at the motel gave us the name and address of the hospital, and our Cuban cabby then drove Dianne and I back to our hotel. When we arrived there, the cabby would not accept any money for his services. He understood how we were trying to help someone in distress; not accepting payment for the fare was his way of helping, too, and we thanked him profusely.

The next day we went to the children's hospital during my lunch break from the medical conference. There we found Frances, looking much better, with Mrs. Patterson and Thomas visiting. Fortunately Frances had not needed to be put on a ventilator thanks to the EMT who had acted quickly enough in giving her the epinephrine and starting her on oxygen. Mrs. Patterson told us that Frances had been started on cortisone and an antibiotic since admission. She was now doing much better, and her mother said she was to be discharged later that afternoon. She once again thanked us profusely for our help the night before. Before we left, I gave Mrs. Patterson one of my business cards. I wrote down for her the name of the hotel and room number where we were staying should they require any further help while in Florida. Several days later, after we had returned to Michigan, we received in the mail a thank you card from the Patterson family in Wisconsin. It was signed by Mr. and Mrs. Patterson, both of whom very much appreciated the help we had provided Frances.

Six years had passed since that fateful night in Florida when we were surprised to receive another communication from the Wisconsin, this time from Frances herself. It was an invitation to her high school graduation along with a letter to us. Frances was the valedictorian of her class. In her letter she said that the theme of her valedictory speech was always try to do your best for others. She told her classmates that the only reason she was alive to give that speech, was because two others had done their best to help her when she almost died from an asthma attack. In the letter she went on to say she was going to college as a pre-medical student. She told us she had been inspired by what we had done for her and wanted to be able to do the same for someone else in her future career in medicine. Sometimes you never know how your actions affect the lives of those you meet.

Christmas

Herman and Liesl, a German couple in their early fifties, lived across the street from us with their youngest, a thirteen year-old son, still at home. Herman was a union carpenter and Liesl a homemaker. They were very good neighbors with an extremely tidy house. Liesl had quite the green thumb with her lawn, flowers, and vegetable garden. Everything was kept immaculate. They had been raised on family farms in a state bordering Canada. To escape the extreme winters they had moved South to work and rear their children. Their two older children, a daughter and elder son, were both out on their own, yet living nearby, so Herman and Liesl still had their family around them.

Unfortunately, as is so often the case, Herman's carpenter union went on strike in early November. He received a very small amount from the strike fund each week, just enough to pay for the simplest of groceries, and they began to deplete their savings just to pay their regular bills. Then one evening in early December, after eating the spicy German sausage with cabbage he loved so much, Herman was in trouble. Within thirty minutes of his meal he had severe unremitting abdominal pain, worse with movement, along with nausea but no vomiting. Liesl called and asked if I would come across the street to see him even though she knew I was not yet licensed to practice medicine. I agreed nonetheless, knowing they could not afford an ER visit at this time unless it was absolutely necessary.

When I entered the living room, I saw Herman sitting very still on the edge of his recliner, holding his right side and sweating, though the room was cool. I had him lie back gently on the recliner so I could examine his abdomen. I found he had right upper quadrant pain, very tender with tapping my fist over the right lower ribs in front, all of which suggested an acute gallbladder attack. It was obvious that Herman needed hospitalization and, most likely, a cholecystectomy, the surgical removal of the gallbladder. Since Liesl couldn't drive, I drove Herman and Liesl to the hospital. He was evaluated by the emergency room doctor with an examination, blood tests, and an ultrasound, then admitted to a surgeon with diagnosis of acute cholecystitis with cholelithiasis - inflammation of the gallbladder with gallstones, respectively. After a few days with no oral intake, IV fluids, and antibiotics, Herman was taken to the operating room and underwent a cholecystectomy.

Gallbladder disease is one of the most common causes of abdominal surgery. Female to male ratio for gallstone disease is 3:1, but both sexes are affected almost equally after age fifty. Age is major risk factor for gallstones and gallbladder disease. In children it is very rare. The use of estrogen is a major risk factor for gallbladder disease. Obesity and fair complexion are also risk factors. An old mnemonic, or memory aid, for gallbladder disease was "female, fat, forty, fertile, and fair". Yet men can also have gallstones and gallbladder disease just as Herman did.

Most gallstones are cholesterol stones. Some are simply pigmented stones while others are a mixture. Herman's were cholesterol stones.

The symptoms caused by gallbladder disease include nausea, vomiting, right upper abdominal pain often radiating to the back, and sometimes abdominal bloating. The pain usually begins fifteen to thirty minutes after a meal, particularly a fatty one. It is rather severe and often constant rather than a true colicky-type pain. The ultrasound may show gallbladder wall thickening and sludge or stones within it. Occasionally, none of these findings will be present on ultrasound. If the clinical findings are highly suggestive of gallbladder disease, the doctor can then order a nuclear medicine scan. For this scan the patient is given a tiny amount of radioactive tracer, which is picked up by the liver and excreted into the bile. Once the radioactive tracer has been injected, the patient is scanned for about the next hour. Then the patient is given an injection of cholecystokinin, a hormone that stimulates the gallbladder to contract. The gallbladder is then scanned again, and the difference in size is calculated. There should be at least 30% or more emptying, the "ejection fraction", of the gallbladder. I have had patients whose ejection fraction was 0%, indicating significant gallbladder disease in spite of having no wall thickening, sludge, or stones on ultrasound.

The usual treatment for an acute gallbladder attack is intravenous fluids, antibiotics for several days, and no oral intake to put the bowel at rest, just as was done in Herman's case. Cholecystectomy is then recommended as it is safer and reduces the total number of hospital days. Nowadays the vast majority of gallbladder surgeries are done through the laparoscope. There are still complicated cases where the old classical open gallbladder surgery must be done, but this is quite uncommon. There is medical therapy available for the dissolution of gallstones, but this is reserved for those with contraindications to either type of surgery. It is effective only about ten percent of the time it is tried.

For Herman this was not a good time to have to have surgery. Their income was very low, and although their health insurance covered most of the expense, they were still responsible for twenty percent of it themselves. This almost exhausted the rest of their savings. Sadly, this all occurred just a few weeks before Christmas. It seemed their family was going to have a very sparse holiday that year.

Knowing all of this, my wife, Dianne, and I decided to provide a little "sneaky" holiday cheer. They would never have accepted a direct gift due to their German pride, but we felt we could get around that. Both of our parents had sent us a little money for Christmas, so we decided to buy them an entire holiday dinner that Christmas Eve, including a turkey, stuffing, mashed potatoes, a gallon of milk, butter, dinner rolls, and vegetables. In the grocery store we happened to spot a display of various recorded tapes.

Dianne picked out a Christmas album by Perry Como for Liesl, and I found a cassette tape of German polkas by Whoopee John for Herman. For their younger son we bought a model airplane, as he enjoyed putting these together. When we got home, we gift-wrapped the three presents, labeling each with their respective names, and writing, "From Santa" on them. That evening we tiptoed across the street and silently placed the items we had purchased on their front porch. Dianne had a nurse friend of hers, whose voice they would not recognize, call to let them know that Santa had been to their house and to check their front porch. Peering from behind our curtains with our lights off, we saw the surprise on their faces when they opened the front door and found the bags with the groceries and presents.

Christmas day we visited Herman and Liesl, ostensibly to see how he was doing after his surgery. Of course, they told us all about the surprise they had found on their front porch. They were very grateful to their anonymous donor for what they had received and explained to us in detail what they had found in the bags of groceries and the presents for each of them. However, both Herman and Liesl knew beyond a doubt that we were not their secret Santa. They were convinced that this had to have been done by someone who knew them from their youth up north. For when they were dating, they danced polkas at barn dances where Whoopee John's band played live, and

Perry Como had been Liesl's favorite singer when she was a teenager.

No, it couldn't have been us.

Colonel

Many years ago, when I was a resident in family practice at the University of Kentucky, there was great competition among OB/GYN residents, family practice residents, and medical students for delivering babies at the University Hospital. For this reason the family practice program had made an arrangement with Appalachian Regional Hospital in Harlan, Kentucky for family practice residents to work a six-week rotation there with Dr. Hurlocker, their OB/GYN attending physician. This would enable us to gain the additional obstetrical experience needed to obtain obstetric privileges once in private practice.

As I planned to do obstetrics in my future practice, I took advantage of this opportunity for two summers in a row. The first time, as we drove to Harlan, we were stunned at the growth of the kudzu. This vine had been imported from Japan by our federal government to be a ground cover for road cuts in the South. Unfortunately, the vine had become invasive, growing up to a foot a day and now devouring over three million acres! We saw it encasing telephone poles, power lines, and even entire houses.

During the two summers we were there, we stayed in an apartment building located between the hospital and a strip mall with a Piggly-Wiggly grocery store. Throughout the first - and most of the second - summer we were there, most of the people of Harlan would speak little or not at all with us. We were outsiders, "not from around here", and the people of Harlan county were very wary of people from the "big city". This was understandable given the history of Harlan County, Kentucky, and how the people had been looked down upon, used, and taken advantage of for decades past. Nonetheless, it made our stay there seem strangely unwelcome.

Not far from the city of Harlan lies the man-made Martin's Fork Lake, where coal companies had trucked in tons of white sand to make a swimming beach for the people of Harlan. We did not go there the first summer we spent in Harlan, but the second summer I had to promise to take our four children swimming at the lake. Several weeks went by, during which I had been very busy with work at the hospital. The morning of July 4th, tired from being on-call the night before, I walked back to the apartment only to have my wife remind me of my promise to take the children swimming. This would be our last opportunity to keep that promise, so on that day we went to the lake.

Though the Martin's Fork Lake is only about fourteen miles from town, it took over a half hour to get there on the twisting, winding mountain road. In addition, huge slow coal trucks often would slow traffic to a crawl. Finally arriving at the lake, we parked our car under the shade of a tree and walked the children down to the beach. We spread out our beach blanket, laid down the towels, and the children took off running to the water's edge. On such a warm day the water felt really cold, so it took them a while to get in, but soon they were "swimming" with delight. Of course the two youngest ones could not really swim, so I had to stay close to them to make sure they would be all right. The older two children were able to swim on their own.

We had been there a few hours enjoying the coolness of the lake in the summer heat when my daughter, our eldest, ran up to me and said, "Daddy, there's a little boy that drowned down the beach!" I replied to her, "Sure. That's not such a funny joke." She insisted, "No really, Daddy! There's a boy that's drowned!". At that point I realized she was in earnest. I had her watch her two youngest brothers and took off running down the beach.

About twenty yards down the beach I saw two men leaning over a little blonde boy lying face down on the sand. He was bluish and not moving. Two men were pushing on his back, then pulling up on his elbows in an attempt to resuscitate him. As I reached them, I said forcefully, "I am a doctor! Let me have him." They immediately stepped aside and let me work.

I turned the boy over on his back and wiped the wet sand off his mouth. I quickly gave him two rescue breaths then checked his carotid pulse; there was none. I immediately gave him a firm "thump" on the chest. Again I checked his pulse, and this time he had one. I then continued giving him mouth-to-mouth resuscitation for a few minutes until he suddenly and spontaneously began to choke and breathe on his own. We sat him up and he vomited what seemed like a gallon of lake water and began crying and shivering. His father, Hank, then wrapped him in a blanket and took him up by their car.

Someone had already called the ambulance to come from the hospital, but it took half an hour for them to arrive. Hank's family had returned to Harlan that summer to visit with his cousin, Jake, who told Hank, "I know all the doctors at the clinic, and he ain't no doctor. You oughta put that boy in your car and drive fast as you can to the hospital!" Hank said nothing, but looked at me with urgent concern in his eyes. He had just seen his son almost die and was scared. I took out my wallet and showed him my Kentucky medical license. I explained to him that I was down for the summer getting extra obstetrical training. I advised Hank not to try to hurry to the hospital. As upset as he was, he was liable to go too fast around a curve and run head-on into a coal truck. I pointed out that his son was breathing, his heart was beating, and although he was frightened and shivering, he was stable. Hank looked at his cousin Jake and said, "I think I'll do what the doctor says."

When the ambulance crew arrived, they were almost shocked to see the young boy sitting up breathing on his own. The driver told me, "Wow! We have a live one! In most cases by the time we get here, the victim is already dead!" They put the young man in their ambulance, covered him with an additional blanket, and began the drive back to Harlan, Hank following in his car, and both going slow enough to be safe. As they left, we decided we'd had enough swimming at the lake that afternoon. We would go back to town ourselves, clean up, and begin preparing our holiday dinner.

After taking a shower to wash off the lake sand, the two youngest boys and I walked over to the hospital to check on the one whose life I had saved. A chest x-ray showed he had aspirated some lake water into his lungs. He had been started on an antibiotic and admitted to be watched for a day or two on the pediatric unit. Again, Hank and his wife thanked me for what I had done, and I assured them I was happy I had the opportunity to be there to help.

We left the hospital and immediately walked across the three parking lots of the hospital, the apartment building, and the Piggly-Wiggly. We went inside to pick out hot-dogs, buns, chips, marshmallows, and a cold watermelon for our Independence Day feast. To my complete surprise, as we pushed our cart up to the cash register to check out, the cashier turned to me and said, "Oh, Dr. Yarbrough! That was a wonderful thing you did out at the lake this afternoon. The people around here really appreciate when someone helps one of their own. We all sure hope you'll come back here to practice. We know you'll be very busy." She kept on talking, saying more than she had in two summers! I couldn't believe how freely she spoke to me, an outsider, or how fast she had found out what happened at the lake. That evening we kept going over what had happened. It was certainly a memorable Fourth of July dinner.

The next day at the hospital, Dr. Hurlocker explained to me that once an outsider like myself had shown such care for one of their own, the people of Harlan would accept them with open arms. This, he said, was why the cashier had spoken to me so openly about what I had done that day. Dr. Hurlocker also confirmed her words that if I were to come back to Harlan, I would have a very busy practice. Unfortunately, I already had made a commitment to go elsewhere and would not be able to do that. Yet after the incident at the lake, it seemed I could go nowhere in town without people thanking me for what I had done. After a while it got to be embarrassing to be thanked so much by so many complete strangers for doing what any decent person should have done in such circumstances.

Weeks later, back at the university, I was called to come to the office of the residency program director. Usually such a call meant there had been some sort of complaint or problem. Naturally, I was quite apprehensive as I entered the director's office, as I had not heard of any problem with my work and could not recall any complaints. As I entered the office, the director stood up and smiled at me. Also in his office was a lady I had never seen before. Apparently, she was from the governor's office and was there to present me with a certificate stating that I had been named an honorary Kentucky Colonel. It seems the mayor of Harlan, with his report to the governor's office about the incident at the lake, had nominated me for this honor. I was speechless.

To this day I still have that framed certificate. Ironically, performing CPR on that little boy was the first time I had ever done so outside of a hospital. So many times we do it in the hospital unsuccessfully, yet when out deep in the countryside, with no equipment of any kind, I was able to save a young boy's life with CPR. Whenever I look at that certificate, I remember that little blonde-haired boy on the beach at Martin's Fork Lake.

Coma

Abigail would not wake up. It had been five days since her gallbladder surgery, and she remained completely unresponsive. There had been no complications with her surgery, and the surgeon had no reason to suspect she would not wake up normally afterward. She had had previous surgeries for which she had been given general anaesthesia without any problems. Sometimes the greatly obese don't wake up right away. General anesthetic agents must be fat soluble to put the brain to sleep, and the anesthetic will leach out of body fat for days after surgery, keeping the patient asleep for a prolonged time. Yet although Abigail was ninety years old, she was not an obese woman. She just would not wake up.

I had first met Abigail two years prior when she came to my office for management of her blood pressure. She had had a very slight stroke in the past but was still able to function quite well. She also had rather advanced osteoarthritis crippling her hands, which limited her ability to sew and crochet, but she was still able to do those things, and they gave her much pleasure. She told me she particularly enjoyed making things for her great grandchildren.

Abigail and her husband had raised seven children on their farm. Widowed for many years, Abigail now lived in a house trailer next to the farmhouse of her son-in-law and eldest daughter. Her daughter checked on her every day, and often they shared meals together. Another of her daughters also lived nearby. Abigail liked having her independence and privacy, and she was comfortable with her living arrangement, especially knowing that help was just across the lawn if she needed it.

Abigail's blood pressure was not hard to control. Indeed, it was well controlled that Saturday afternoon then she suddenly developed acute abdominal pain with low-grade fever, nausea, and vomiting. Her daughter took her immediately to the emergency room. On examination I found she was tender over the upper right quadrant of the abdomen, the gallbladder area, and I felt she was having an acute gallbladder attack. I obtained an ultrasound of her abdomen which showed her gallbladder to be full of stones with a thickened wall. These changes were consistent with an acute gallbladder attack, known as acute cholecystitis. I admitted her to the regular medical floor, began her on IV fluids, medication for the nausea, an antibiotic and pain medicine, and consulted one of our local surgeons. He agreed with my initial stabilizing treatment, and two days later he took her to the operating room for removal of her gallbladder, a cholecystectomy. Most patients undergoing this kind of surgery awaken after a short time in recovery. She did not.

Her daughters were concerned, as was I, that there may have been some type of neurologic occurrence during surgery. On the second day of her coma I ordered a CT scan of the brain to see if she had suffered another stroke, intracranial bleed, or other finding that might explain the coma. However, her CT scan was essentially unchanged from the one obtained at the time of her stroke several years before. There were no new findings that might have explained her coma. Both the surgeon and I were at a loss to understand why she was not waking up.

For five days after surgery the nursing staff would bathe her each day, turn her every two hours, and keep her IV fluid running to maintain adequate hydration. Yet through all this Abigail showed no response of any kind. Indeed, the nurses reported she had no response even when her Foley urinary catheter had to be changed. Abigail remained a mystery. The morning of the fifth day postoperative day, when I went into her room to see Abigail, I found the surgeon already there, talking to her two eldest daughters. I positioned myself on the opposite side of her bed and listened. He explained to the daughters, who had durable power of attorney for Abigail's health care, that sometimes we have to just "let go". He advised that we stop all treatment and allow her to die peacefully in the coma. Abigail's daughters seemed to be accepting of this and had a look of resignation on their faces.

I was not ready to quit yet. I suggested we could try a massive dose of Solu-Medrol, an injectable cortisone agent. This could be given intravenously over an hour's time. If Abigail had suffered any kind of swelling of the brain, or cerebral edema, this might reverse it and bring her out of the coma. When I mentioned this, the surgeon shrugged his shoulders, remarking, "You're asking for a miracle." I looked at him and responded, "Well, you know, sometimes you get one." He shrugged again and left the room with the two daughters following, as they had a few more questions for him.

I then performed my examination of Abigail. Her lungs showed no pneumonia, fluid, or congestion, and she was still breathing well on her own. The nurses had reported she would occasionally cough on her own, too. Her heart was beating regularly, and she had no skin breakdown of any kind on her back or buttocks. Bed sores are a major risk to patients in her condition, but she showed no signs of developing one. Unfortunately, she was still not responsive to touch, voice, or even slight pinprick.

After completing my examination, I went to the nurses station to write up my note on her for that day. While I was writing, her eldest daughter came up to me and asked, "What was that medicine you were talking about? Is it toxic or expensive?" I explained to her the nature of Solu-Medrol, a rapid but short acting cortisone preparation, that was given intravenously. The usual dose would be 250 mg. By giving Abigail 1,000 mg I thought we might bring her out of the coma. Of course, there was no guarantee it would work, but I felt it was worth a try since Abigail had nothing to lose at this point, and the medication was not expensive. She went to talk with her sister for a few minutes. Together they came back and said, "We would like you to try that medicine for our mother." I advised them I would do so and ordered the Solu-Medrol to be given that morning.

All through that day there was no change in Abigail's condition. Well into the evening there was still no change, so her daughters went home. However, at 7 a.m. the following morning, when the nurses aide came in to take her blood pressure, Abigail suddenly opened her eyes, sat bolt upright in the bed, and said, "When is breakfast around here? I'm hungry!" At this the nurses aide screamed and ran out of the room to find the nurse. She, too, was shocked to see Abigail sitting up and talking. She called me right away with the good news.

By the time I arrived to make rounds, Abigail was sitting up on the side of the bed, eating her breakfast and talking up a storm with her daughters. As I came into the room, Abigail greeted me with, "Good morning, Doctor!" It was obvious that she was fully aware of her surroundings. She knew that she had been in the hospital and had gallbladder surgery, but she was startled to learn that she had been "asleep" for five days. Her daughters seemed even more startled to see their mother sitting up eating breakfast and talking as if nothing had happened.

Apparently my hunch had been correct. Abigail had suffered some degree of cerebral edema due to the anesthesia and surgery, brain swelling that was reversed by the Solu-Medrol. A few hours later the surgeon came by to see her. The nurses told me later that the shock on his face was priceless. The following day I discharged Abigail with follow-up appointments for her with the surgeon and with me.

For the next seven years I took care of Abigail, making sure we kept her blood pressure under good control to prevent another stroke. After that her daughters convinced her to change doctors as I was no longer a "preferred provider" for her insurance. I'm not sure if she is still living. She would now be over one-hundred years old if she is. What happened to her after the gallbladder surgery and her remarkable recovery with Solu-Medrol is one of the best memories I have in my thirty years of family medicine. For that one time, at least, we got our miracle.

Complete

Sometimes there can be a marked disconnect between the terms a physician uses, as opposed to the patient's understanding of those same terms. Each person in such a case has a very clear understanding of what the particular words mean to them, yet such understandings may not be congruent. Even what may seem like the simplest of words can create serious confusion. Perhaps one of the most common instances of this relates to the word "complete".

To the layman the phrase "complete hysterectomy" means the surgical removal of the uterus, both fallopian tubes, and both ovaries, all in one operation. However, in past decades a doctor might have performed a supracervical hysterectomy, namely, removing only the upper portion of the uterus while leaving the lower portion intact. This was not uncommonly done as a last resort in cases of severe uterine bleeding to stop the hemorrhaging. That operation was called a "partial hysterectomy" by the doctor, indicating removal of only part of the uterus. The term "complete hysterectomy" back then referred to the removal of the entire uterus, but not the fallopian tubes or ovaries.

The medical term for what the layman knows as "complete hysterectomy" would be a total hysterectomy with bilateral salpingectomy and oophorectomy, the latter terms referring to the removal of the fallopian tubes and ovaries, respectively. This disconnect in understanding drastically affected a patient of mine, Louise. Apparently, at age forty-two in 1962, she underwent removal of her uterus for abnormal bleeding. When she asked the doctor if he had done a complete hysterectomy, he told her he had done so. She took this to mean that he removed her tubes and ovaries as well, but that was not the doctor's understanding of the words she had used. Since she began having hot flashes and other menopausal symptoms within six months, she simply assumed that her ovaries were gone. They were not.

Not long after I had moved to Kansas, I became Louise's doctor when she was a seventy-four year old widow. I treated her for several years for the very common triad of diabetes type II, high cholesterol, and hypertension. I prescribed her medications for each of these problems, and she was doing quite well on them. She always agreed to her annual mammogram but not a pelvic examination, saying, "They took all that out years ago." So for several years her care was rather routine.

One evening, however, after a chicken dinner with her children, she awoke at 4 a.m. with severe cramping abdominal pain, progressively worsening and finally causing nausea and vomiting. She called me about the pain, and I advised her to go to the ER where I would meet her. On examination I found she had severe central abdominal tenderness but no definite mass that I could feel. Initial x-rays of her abdomen, along with her symptoms, suggested mechanical ileus, or non-functioning bowel due to physical obstruction. She also had an abnormally elevated white blood cell count, and she could not tell me if she had had an appendectomy with her "complete hysterectomy" forty years prior. Since acute appendicitis is still the most common cause of acute surgical abdomen in adult patients, I consulted one of our local surgeons.

The surgeon examined her and felt she had adhesions from her old surgery causing bowel obstruction. Adhesions are white scar tissues, often like a spider's web, that can entrap a loop or segment of bowel and cause obstruction. They are believed to be caused by inflammation of the lining of the bowels due to the "trauma" of surgery, though no one really knows why some people form adhesions after an operation and others do not. Sometimes they can form right away and cause immediate problems, while at other times the patient can go for decades without trouble until suddenly the bowel obstructs. The surgeon agreed she needed surgery, and with her consent he took her to the operating room.

In surgery she was found to have extensive filmy white adhesions throughout her abdomen, some of which had entrapped a loop of her jejunum, the first portion of the small intestine past the duodenum.

However, the surgeon also found a small tumor on her ileum, the last portion of her small intestine. He removed the involved segment of her ileum and performed an end-to-end anastomosis, a reconnection of the cut ends of the bowel. He also removed some of the lymph nodes draining the resected bowel. Finally, he noted that she had, indeed, had her appendix removed during her old operation.

Postoperatively, Louise had some problems with fluid retention and low sodium. With these corrected she recovered well from her surgery and was discharged home. However, the pathology report on the surgical tissue specimen identified an adenocarcinoma, a form of cancer, the origin of which could not be determined. In other words, the pathologist was not certain which organ had become cancerous. Yet due to the location of the tumor, the surgeon and the cancer specialist, to whom the patient was referred, both assumed this was a tumor of the small intestine. The oncologist treated her accordingly with what seemed to be the appropriate chemotherapy, and she tolerated the treatments quite well. Unfortunately, it also caused her to develop a fine tremor which annoyed her considerably. As she put it laughingly, "I can't eat peas with a knife any more."

For the next four years there was no evidence of recurrence of the disease. I still saw Louise regularly for her blood pressure, cholesterol, and diabetes. She also saw her oncologist twice a year. During this time she never again developed problems from adhesions. However, one day she came to my office with complaints of pelvic pain and pressure. She thought she might be having a bladder infection. To her surprise, her urine examination was entirely normal. On physical examination, though, she had an apparent mass in the lower abdomen extending down into the pelvis. I ordered a CT scan of abdomen and pelvis which showed large bilateral irregular masses filling her pelvis.

I immediately referred Louise to a gynecologist. She was able to get Louise to agree to a pelvic exam which confirmed our suspicions. The gynecologist then made arrangements with the general surgeon to work together to remove the tumor masses. Once again, now over eighty, Louise underwent general anesthesia and surgery. Two separate irregular masses, each the size of a baby's head, were found and removed. The masses proved to be cancers of Louise's left and right ovaries, organs which Louise had thought were removed over forty years before! In retrospect both the surgeon and the gynecologist now felt that the adenocarcinoma previously removed from the ileum may also have been ovarian in origin.

Once again Louise underwent staging and chemotherapy, this time for ovarian cancer, and once again she tolerated the treatment quite well, especially considering her age. I continued seeing her for her other medical problems until at age ninety-two she changed doctors, as I was no longer on her insurance. Since then I have learned she finally passed away at age ninety-six, from "old age", fifty-six years after her "complete" hysterectomy! Some misunderstandings can last a long time.

Confidentiality

Some of the laws we have in this country can be very destructive of family life. Certainly there is the well-known example of what welfare laws have done to destroy black family life, so that now almost three-fourths of all black babies in this country are born to unwed mothers. Yet those of all races have suffered violence to family life due to misguided laws relating to so-called confidentiality for minors regarding matters related to sexual activity. The excuse for such laws is that minors will not seek medical care for sexually transmitted diseases or pregnancy if their parents might find out about it.

These confidentiality laws build a "wall of separation" between minor children and their parents, the very people those children need the most and who love them the most. Such laws can often cause more harm than good. Suicide is now the third leading cause of death among teenagers in this country according to "Morbidity and Mortality among U.S. Adolescents", a study published in the American Journal of Public Health in 1996. One wonders how many of those deaths could have been prevented if these children had confided in their parents. Depression is especially prevalent among sexually active teenagers, according to the "National Longitudinal Survey of Adolescent Health", also published in 1996. Finally, the "National Campaign to Prevent Teen Pregnancy", published in June of 2000, surveyed sexually active teenagers, the majority of whom reported they wished they had waited longer or never started having sexual relations.

Given these findings, it is not surprising that most responsible physicians will urge underage minors to talk with their parents about what is going on in their lives so they can get the advice and support they need from those who care the most about them. While not all parents respond in a loving manner in such situations, confidentiality laws take the decision and judgment away from the doctor and the patient, so that the most loving parent-child relationships are the ones most harmed by these same laws.

I would like to relate to you just two of the many examples of the foolishness of such laws I have seen during my thirty years of family practice. The first involved a young girl who had been sexually active and had missed her last two menstrual periods. She came to my office worried she might be pregnant, and she told me she knew that state laws prevented my telling her parents about her visit. I obtained a pregnancy test on her which was indeed positive. She was clearly ten weeks along with this pregnancy, given the results of her examination and date of her last menstrual period. I asked her if she would not talk with her mother about this, as she seemed very anxious and wanted help to decide what to do. She had not yet talked to her mother and was afraid to do so. I pointed out to her, however, that her mother probably already knew that she was pregnant and was just waiting for her daughter to confide in her.

Astounded, she could not understand how that could possibly be. I asked her who emptied the trash cans in the bathroom; she replied that was done by her mother. I then asked her who purchased the groceries for the family; again she said her mother did that task. Finally, I asked her if she thought her mother was so stupid as not to notice that her daughter had not been using feminine hygiene products for the last two months. Her eyes opened wide and her jaw dropped, as she suddenly realized her mother was, indeed, probably aware of her predicament. She assured me she would go home that night and talk with her mother about her situation. The following week she returned with her mother to begin her prenatal care. She told me she had been surprised to find how supportive her parents were in spite of what mistakes she may have made. She thanked me for having urged her to talk with her parents.

The second case involved a sixteen year-old girl whose parents were divorced. As is so often the case in divorce, this young teenage girl desperately needed the presence of a father figure in her life. Sadly, this desire often leads such girls to turn for male attention and affection to young men whose hormones lead them to take advantage. This particular girl had been sexually active with two different boys. Her mother found out and brought her in for an examination to rule out any sexual transmitted disease or pregnancy. I discussed this with the daughter, and she was willing to have this done. We obtained the necessary specimens and were able to assure her that there was no evidence so far that she had contracted HIV, gonorrhea, Chlamydia, HPV, syphilis, hepatitis B, or other sexually transmitted diseases. Moreover, her pregnancy test was negative.

We sent the bill for her care to her mother. She then forwarded it to the girl's father, who lived in another town but was responsible for his daughter's medical bills until she was of age. Not long after we had sent the bill in the mail, we received a phone call from this girl's father. He wanted an explanation for why his daughter had this bill for medical care and laboratory testing. He explained that he was worried about what was going on with her. He had worked hard to maintain a close relationship with her and had visitation with her at certain times of the year. He assured us they had a good relationship, and he was concerned about his daughter's well-being.

Unfortunately, due to the confidentiality laws mentioned above, we were technically not allowed to explain to this concerned father what had been done and why it was necessary. This caring father was clearly still an active part of his daughter's life, but we were not permitted by law to tell him anything about his daughter's care. He started to became very irate on the telephone and insisted that he had to know why this medical care was necessary, and these costs incurred, if he was going to pay the bill.

My office nurse, thinking quickly on her feet, then explained to the father that there were state laws prohibiting the release to parents of information regarding sexually transmitted disease screening or pregnancy testing for a minor child. She asked if he knew that there were such laws, and, very mollified, he softly replied that he did. My nurse then told him that because of such legislation, she was not able to tell him about the services his daughter had been given. After a long pause, the father replied, "I will be sending a check for the full amount of this bill. Thank you very much for what you have not told me. I will be contacting my daughter soon to have a heart-to-heart talk with her."

I found out later that this girl did have a long talk with her father, and with the recent scare she had about STDs or pregnancy, she made the decision to remain chaste thereafter until she was married. Her father and mother were both pleased with this decision, and their daughter felt relieved to not have to deal with the peer pressure to be sexually active again. I still wonder if she had not confided in her parents, whether she would have made such a decision otherwise. In case you are wondering, she remained true to her decision in the years that followed. She has now been happily married for several years and has two children of her own.

Depression

When I first saw Isabel about 10 years ago, she was a seventy year-old woman, tall and thin, with short bushy gray hair and piercing ice-blue eyes. She came to see me because her legs were swollen, or in her words, "turning to concrete". She had previously seen another doctor who had done her hysterectomy for cancer followed by radium implants, but she had failed to keep followup visits with him after several years. When she went to him about the swelling, he "scolded" her for not having returned sooner, so she walked out on him, deciding never to return. This was a sensitive time for her, as her husband had passed away earlier that year, and she was just getting used to being alone. She had worked most of her life to help support the family, but now at her age she was no longer able to work. All four of her children had moved far away, and her friends at church were her main emotional support now.

On examination I found she had a dense, brawny edema (swelling) in both legs extending up almost to the groin. Her skin was very firm to the touch but without discoloration or oozing of fluid. Remarkably, her chest was completely clear of congestive fluid, and her heart had a good strong beat without irregularity or murmur. She walked with a shuffling gait with trouble bending her knees and ankles due to the swelling. Before she left the office, I obtained blood for thyroid testing, since hypothyroidism could cause this kind of swelling, and a CAT scan of her abdomen and pelvis. With her previous history of uterine cancer and this massive swelling, there was certainly the possibility of a recurrent pelvic tumor blocking venous return from the legs and thus causing the edema. Finally, I had her get a blood count since she looked pale.

Upon her return four days later, Isabel told me she had been prayed over repeatedly through her church and felt she was getting better. She said she felt the Lord was "purging" her body of something that shouldn't have been there. She thought her legs were more flexible now. However, on examination I did not find any change in her legs. Except for anemia with low iron, her blood tests were normal. The CT scan of her abdomen and pelvis was also normal. I started Isabel on Lasix, a potent diuretic, to eliminate the excess fluid and referred her for upper gastrointestinal endoscopy and a colonoscopy. These tests were important as common causes of anemia in her age group are colon cancer or ulcer. Fortunately, both endoscopies were normal. When she returned to me, her legs were dramatically better with just a trace of edema at her ankles. She now could bend her knees and ankles easily, and her gait had returned to normal. However, she appeared to be rather depressed but would not admit to it. She insisted she would continue to improve through prayer alone. Due to her anemia, I had her start an iron supplement and asked her to return in three months for recheck.

Unfortunately, with the relief of the swelling in her legs, she began walking much faster. Early that autumn she tripped on the sidewalk in front of her house and broke her leg. Since she lived alone, she had to be admitted to a nursing home for rehabilitation with the expectation that she would return to her own home after her rehab was complete. I continued to see her at the nursing home, and during this time she seemed more depressed. I felt this was due to her being in the nursing home, and that this would likely improve when she went home. I again discussed medication for depression, and again she flatly refused it. She insisted she would do better when she was home.

Unfortunately, after Isabel was discharged home, she did not keep her follow-up visit with me. I tried to call her, but there was no answer at her house. I heard next from her pastor. He had gone to see her at the house since she had stopped coming to church. He told me he felt she was extremely depressed and would benefit from an antidepressant medication. I tended to agree with this judgment, but I advised him that we could not force her to take a pill for depression; she had to agree to do so. It would do no good to prescribe medication she wouldn't take. He understood and promised me he would visit with her again and try once more to convince her to accept treatment for depression.

Her pastor tried calling Isabel several more times, but she would not answer the telephone. He finally decided to return to her house. It was early winter and very cold. No one would answer the door. Worried about her, he peeked in her windows and spotted her legs on the floor extending beyond the sofa. He called the police who came and forced open the front door. They found her barely conscious, lying on the living room floor. The police officer called for an ambulance, and she was taken to the emergency room. There she was found to be hypothermic and dehydrated. Her heart was racing with a pulse of 120 and her core temperature was only 97.6°. Gradually warmed and rehydrated, she became more alert. She recognized me and realized she was in a hospital, but she did not know the date, day of the week, or what year it was. She was admitted and her home medication resumed.

The next morning her nurse reported that Isabel had eaten very little and was throwing things at the staff, yelling for them to get her out. When I went to her room, she was fully alert but completely disoriented. Shaking with fear, her eyes wide open, she screamed at me to get her out of the hospital right away as her bed was on fire, the flames flickering all around her. She then began to ask other people - who were not there - to help her. It was obvious that she would need urgent psychiatric treatment. Now her care began to be much more complicated.

None of her four children lived nearby, nor did any of them have durable power of attorney for health care for Isabel. She had no advanced directives permitting any of them to direct her care. Given this, I called the county attorney to get a court order remanding her to a nearby psychiatric program that specialized in treating the elderly. He advised me we would have to have the county mental health services evaluate her first. I contacted them, and they came that very morning. The psychologist who saw her concurred that she needed urgent psychiatric hospital admission. We were then able to get the court order to effect her transfer to the psychiatric facility.

Unfortunately, one of her daughters, living over three-hundred miles away, found out about her mother's condition and insisted that we merely start her on antidepressant pills and send her home. I explained to the daughter that this would not be appropriate since the medication takes weeks to begin working, not a matter of hours, and that her mother was hallucinating, delusional, and at risk of harming herself. Her present condition warranted inpatient management. The daughter refused to allow her mother to be transferred to the psychiatric facility, but I informed her that in the absence of a document showing she had durable power-of-attorney for healthcare, her mother would be transferred. She replied to me, "We'll see about that. You're going to regret ever interfering with my decisions!" She called her attorney and complained to our hospital administrator, but she quickly found out that I was right.

Transferring Isabel to the psychiatric facility ultimately saved her life. The psychiatrist there recognized the severity of her depression and tried her on several medications, none of which seemed to help. She would not eat or come out of her room. Finally, before resorting to electroconvulsive therapy, ECT, as a last resort, he tried the combination of Cymbalta and Wellbutrin. Together these two medicines began to lift her depression. She started eating and drinking and began to socialize with the other patients and staff. Over the next few weeks she improved so much that she could be discharged back to the nursing home where she had been with her broken leg. I talked with her psychiatrist before the transfer back. He informed me if Cymbalta and Wellbutrin had not worked, she would have to have had ECT.

ECT has gotten a bad reputation from false representations of it on television and in movies. In ECT the patient is given general anesthesia plus a paralyzing medication and connected to an EEG machine. There is thus no indication they are having a seizure from the electric shock except for the changes in the brain wave pattern on the EEG. Unlike antidepressant medications, which take weeks to work, ECT relieves depression immediately. The only side effect of consequence from ECT is spotty permanent memory loss when the patient awakens. However, with a life-threatening depression such as Isabel's, electroshock therapy can be lifesaving and worth the risk. Later I found out from one of her sons that several family members had had severe depression, some committing suicide, and one had undergone ECT.

Once back at the nursing home Isabel settled in and adjusted well. She was pleased to find other residents still there with whom she had been friends during her previous stay. What really cheered her was learning that her pastor had arranged for the church van to pick her up each week for services. After two months at the nursing home, Isabel decided to sell her house and live out the rest of her days there. She appreciated not having to do the housecleaning, cooking, and washing, or pay for taxes, insurance, and maintenance on the house. She is still living at the nursing home. As severe as her depression was, and as difficult as it was to bring under control, I will never change or stop her medicines. She agrees she wants to continue them, for she never again wants to see people or flames that aren't there!

Emphysema

Lorna Nash was not an attractive woman. Short and stocky, her figure resembled that of an oak tree. Her arms and legs were thin with flaking, powdery-dry skin. She wore her hair - stringy, deep brown, and tinged with gray, straight and long, almost to her waist, or where her waist should be. Her complexion had the blotchy, dried orange peel appearance of one who had smoked too many packs of cigarettes for too many years. Her voice was always hoarse due to the puffy swelling of the vocal cords so common in heavy smokers. She usually wore a dark flowered sack dress and house slippers. Lorna was one of those from whom the well-off would automatically avert their gaze when passing in a store.

Lorna had not been to a doctor in many years, certainly not since the death of her husband, Steve, from a heart attack five years before. They had been married for almost forty years before he passed away. Steve had worked hard all his life but, unfortunately, never did save much money. He also left her with neither a pension nor life insurance. They did have one daughter, but she lived several states away and rarely communicated with Lorna. I suspected she was embarrassed by her mother. Lorna still smoked over a pack a day and had hypertension. Once, when her breathing became really labored, she finally agreed to let her neighbor, a long-time patient of mine, bring her to my office.

When Lorna arrived, the nurse took her to an examining room right away as Lorna was so short of breath. Her blood pressure was quite high, and she was working very hard to breathe. On examination that first time her face was perspiring and slightly bluish. Her chest showed markedly increased diameter with severe expiratory wheezing throughout. Lorna had rather poor air exchange in spite of her straining to breathe. She also had slight swelling in her ankles due to cor pulmonale. This condition is caused by the abnormal emphysematous architecture of the lungs from years of smoking. This creates markedly elevated pressure in the pulmonary vessels. As a result, blood flow backs up in the right side of the heart, ultimately causing swelling in the feet and legs. Surprisingly, although Lorna was extremely short of breath, she was still somewhat able to talk. After all these years of medical practice, I still find it remarkable how dramatically the body can adapt to ever-worsening physiologic conditions.

In addition to starting her on supplemental oxygen, we began Lorna right away on a nebulizer inhalation treatment with albuterol, a bronchodilator medication. This medication is also available as metered dose inhaler or "puffer", but those devices generate a fine spray or mist. The nebulizer machine, on the other hand, generates a fine cloud or fog of medication. The smaller a particle is, the deeper it can get into the chest. Thus the nebulizer delivery system is much more effective than a metered-dose inhaler.

Within twenty minutes Lorna was breathing much better. She was now able to talk much more effectively and told me she had been coughing up more mucus, which now was yellow and green; normally it was gray or white. I prescribed her an inexpensive generic antibiotic as well as albuterol for her to use in a nebulizer machine. Since she could not afford to rent or purchase her own machine, we loaned her our spare office machine until she got better. Before she left, we also gave her a long-acting cortisone shot to relieve the inflammation in her airways and help suppress the wheezing. I asked her to call back in two days to tell us how she was doing. Before she left, she paid five dollars on her bill.

Office calls for five dollars had disappeared long before Lorna was born. At the time she came to the office, an office call would range from $95 to $115. As we got to know Lorna better, we knew it would not be possible for her to afford the usual office fees. Her five dollars was like the "widow's mite", all she could afford. I would have accepted this as payment in full in her case, except that I had signed Medicare and private insurance contracts. These contracts specifically stated in a "most-favored nation" clause that their members could not be charged more than anyone else for the same service. There was never an exception made for the poor, so according to these contracts, I could not charge Lorna less for an office call. This was true of Medicare, Blue Cross/Blue Shield, Aetna,

United Health Care, Cigna, and nearly all other insurance contracts.

However, we devised a way around this problem. For patients like Lorna, who could not afford a regular office fee, we could charge the full amount, then later write off as "uncollectable" most of the charge. This was the "work-around" technique we used in Lorna's case. I would average seeing her four or five times a year for blood pressure checks and for acute episodes of lung disease. Each time we would charge her the full price for her office calls, and each time she was faithful in making payments of $5. Of course, she would never get her bill paid off, but we didn't mind. Each year at Easter we would write off $500 or more from her bill and catch her up! This technique kept me from getting in trouble with the insurance companies and Medicare, while still permitting us to help those in need.

One summer Lorna had gone several months without an office call. After her Easter write-off she was close to getting her account paid off when she became ill again. We saw her right away, since with a delay of even a few days, she could get sick enough to have to be hospitalized. As she was checking out at the front desk, she remarked, "Why is it I always seem to get sick just before I get my bill paid off?" The nurse replied without missing a beat, "Because you just get lonely and need to come see us!" Lorna began laughing. The nurse went on, "Besides - having a bill to pay off gives you a reason to keep on living!" Lorna then had to sit down - she was laughing so hard!

Over the six years I took care of Lorna, we got to know each other very well. We learned over time that Lorna was a very generous and kind person. Though she had little, she would give much. She was always concerned more about others and how they were doing, always try to help wherever she could. Limited as her resources were, Lorna would prepare funeral meals for families in her church who had lost loved ones. She also would take meals and whatever household items she could spare to those recovering from a house fire. In short, though not a physically attractive woman, she was a beautiful person.

Unfortunately, we a received call one day from her neighbor to let us know that Lorna had died. She had had a massive stroke during the night and was found dead in her bed by the neighbor the next morning. In a way this was a blessing. She had passed from this life in her sleep without having to struggle with the end-stage suffocation of advanced emphysema. Lorna reminded us all of a very important lesson - not to judge others by their appearance. We wrote off her final bill.

Fraud

How many times I have heard someone complain about fraud and abuse in Medicare and Medicaid! Hardly a month goes by that some politician or other doesn't complain loudly to the media about tax dollars wasted by fraud and abuse in these programs. The federal government has introduced program after program over the years to detect fraud and abuse, so that now I suspect they are spending as much to detect and stop fraud as they are losing from it, for the overwhelming majority of doctors are honest and doing their best to care for the patients who must rely on those programs for their health care.

I, myself, was once accused of abuse in the Medicare program years ago when I practiced in Michigan. One day I received a call from an investigator at the Detroit offices of the Medicare carrier. She told me that since I had been ordering mammograms on my patients of Medicare age, I had to refund all the money I collected for those tests. I told the investigator I collected no money for mammograms but just scheduled them to be done at our hospital's certified mammogram unit. Also, I reminded her of all the then-recent media articles complaining that doctors didn't order mammograms enough. Finally, I explained to her the American Cancer Society recommendations for breast cancer screening. I pointed out to her that I was following those accepted standards of care. She then told me that because mammograms were not at that time a covered procedure under Medicare, their office considered them medically unnecessary. To this day I still don't know how I was expected to pay back funds never paid for mammograms that Medicare didn't cover anyway! That was the first and last time I have ever been accused of fraud or abuse. Not many years before that, though, I had seen real fraud up close.

At the time, I was just out of residency and trying to establish my first practice. The hospital was twenty-six miles away, where I was the newest and least experienced physician on the medical staff. Only ten miles down the road, on the rural highway outside of town, was the office of another physician, consisting of two double-wide trailers set side-by-side in a gravel parking lot. Whenever I drove past this office on my way to the hospital, I always saw at least a dozen or more cars parked there with a steady flow of people going in and out. This same doctor had once sat next to me at a medical staff meeting, telling me how large his practice was, how he saw over sixty patients a day, and how he was going to retire a millionaire by age forty-five. At the time I brushed off his words as braggadocio and a crude attempt to intimidate a new physician, struggling to build his practice. Later I would find he had told me the truth.

After I had been there about six months, this other physician came down with appendicitis and had to have surgery. As he had no partner, I was asked by the chief of the medical staff if I would care for his patients currently hospitalized for the next two days. He said he was asking me as I was new, not yet very busy, and could handle the extra work. I agreed, figuring that helping out a colleague might win me the respect of other doctors on staff. The chief of staff seemed very relieved when I agreed, apparently because - as I found out later - every other physician on staff had refused.

I obtained a roster of the patients that other doctor had admitted and was shocked to see that his patients accounted for almost half the hospital's occupancy. As I began reviewing some of their charts at the nurses' station, my eyes were opened. The first chart I read was that of a woman in her mid-fifties with alleged severe abdominal pain, vomiting, and fever, who had been admitted three days prior. The history and physical examination dictated by her doctor was quite detailed and gave the impression this woman was quite ill. He had ordered multiple blood tests and x-ray examinations on her, yet they all had come back essentially normal. When I went to her room to talk with this patient, I found that nothing she told me about herself and the reason for her admission matched with what had been dictated into her chart. Though the history and physical and all the progress notes seemed thorough and well-documented, none of it was true.

At first I thought I might have entered the wrong room and been talking to the wrong patient, but she assured me that she was the individual whose name was on the front of the chart in my hand. Yet what was recorded in her chart did not match what she was telling me. She told me she never had fever, vomiting, or severe abdominal pain but just a mild stomach ache for which she had gone to the doctor. She had been feeling tired lately, so she had no objection to spending a few days in the hospital while someone else would take care of her children and do the housework. Her history and physical said that she had eight children, but she told me she had only five. The notes said that two others in her household had also been sick with this, but she told me she was the only one ill in her whole family. She was also surprised that I was spending so much time with her, yet I had only been in the room about ten minutes. This turned out to be the case with every one of that doctor's patients I saw that day in the hospital. I quickly learned I could not rely on the accuracy of anything that had been dictated in the chart. I tried to do the best I could by these patients, sorting out truth from fiction. I wrote my notes in their charts and drove home.

Later I found out how he managed to "see" sixty patients a day. A patient with high blood pressure would come to his office, checked in at the front desk, and immediately be taken to one of the exam rooms by his nurse. The nurse would visit with the patient a few minutes, check their blood pressure, and then fill out a prescription to renew their medication for only one week. The chart with the new prescription was then put in a pocket by the door. The doctor would come by, say hello, scribble a quick note, sign the prescription, and have the patient come back again in one week. He was then onto the next room, having spent about sixty seconds with each patient. During that time he recorded in each chart a brief but fictitious examination, one that he had never done. It was with this system that he could "see" so many people each day. He billed Medicaid for each weekly visit; over 95% of his practice was Medicaid.

I resolved that I would report this man to State and federal investigators, but a more experienced physician, whom I trusted, advised me against it. He told me this physician had twice been investigated by the state for possible Medicaid fraud, having been reported by two different colleagues. Yet the state never brought charges of fraud against him, for his charts seemed to document proper care, though it was care his patients had never received. Moreover, somehow he found out who had reported him and then brought lawsuits for defamation of character against them. Although these lawsuits would not be successful, they still cost the other physicians a great deal of time and money. My experienced colleague rightly warned me that I could not afford to defend myself from him at that point in my career. It was frustrating to be unable to stop this dishonest physician, but at least I had had the opportunity to see Medicaid fraud up close and in detail. I also knew that I would never again agree to cover for that physician no matter who asked me to do it.

The last I heard was that physician had indeed retired a millionaire by age forty-five and had left the country. I had also moved on, fortunate that I would never again have to deal that kind of medical care. I don't know if the procedures and practices instituted by Medicare and Medicaid in the twenty-five years since then have been successful in eliminating this type of "Medicaid mill", but I sincerely hope that they have. One thing hasn't changed, though. I still follow the American Cancer Society guidelines for mammograms.

Hair Ball

Ralph was an imposing man, six feet three inches tall and weighing 250 pounds, with half-closed slate-blue eyes and a huge gray Fu Man Chu mustache. He had been going bald for several years, and like so many men who are losing their scalp hair, Ralph was unconsciously compensating for his loss with the growth and maintenance of facial hair. In Ralph's case his mustache was quite large, long, and never trimmed. Ralph worked as a cross-country truck driver, an occupation he had pursued for decades, long before his hair began falling out. Like most truck drivers, Ralph was not in the habit of eating a healthy diet. As a result he had develop gallstones and previously had a cholecystectomy, removal of the gallbladder along with associated gallstones.

Ralph initially came in to see me about chronic abdominal discomfort. For two years Ralph had had intermittent epigastric discomfort, a pain located in the upper central abdomen just under the rib margins. He had been treating himself for this with Tums, but this was not very effective. He then switched to over-the-counter Tagamet which at first seemed to be effective, but it also lost its effectiveness over time. Ralph then saw another doctor who listened to his story and prescribed prescription Prilosec. Once again, this had seemed to help for a while, but then it, too, lost its effectiveness. Now in addition to indigestion and acid reflux symptoms, Ralph was complaining of a chronic stomach discomfort, a feeling of fullness, worse after just a few bites of a meal. He denied any blood loss symptoms and claimed that his bowels were normal. On examination, I found that Ralph had a fullness in the epigastric area, a football sized mass that was mobile and quite firm. This indicated to me that Ralph's problem was not just due to simple indigestion, acid reflux, or even ulcer. It was something more seriously wrong, and my initial thought was a tumor. Given these findings, I scheduled Ralph for an upper GI x-ray. This showed clearly a football-sized bezoar, an extremely rare finding.

A bezoar is a mass trapped in the stomach, contents of which can be quite variable. Bezoar comes from a Persian word which means antidote, and animal bezoars in ancient times were thought to be a universal antidote to poisons and were highly sought after. A glass of water containing a bezoar had to be drunk by the person who is poisoned in order to supposedly cure him. One would think the cure was worse than the disease, and of course, the cure was never successful.

As in Ralph's case a trichobezoar is essentially a human hair ball. It develops from eating or chewing on hair. It is believed that the trichobezoar forms because hair is so long and smooth that it cannot be pushed forward with normal peristalsis, or contractions of the stomach. In Ralph's case it was apparent that he had developed the habit of chewing on his mustache. I even witnessed him doing this when he was in my office. Most of the time a trichobezoar is seen in young girls with long hair who have a nervous habit of chewing on their hair. Hairs breaks off and accumulate in the stomach, forming a giant hair ball. In addition to human hair, a bezoar can be formed from undigested food, called a phytobezoar. An extreme high-fiber diet is felt to be a risk factor for a phytobezoar, particularly if the patient has had previous gastric surgery with removal of part of the stomach. There is also a lactobezoar that has been seen in premature babies on formula feedings.

The usual symptoms of a bezoar are those that Ralph was experiencing, namely, stomach acidity, upper abdominal pain, indigestion, and fullness after meals. In severe cases there can be bleeding of the stomach or complete intestinal obstruction needing prompt surgical treatment. There can even be death of the bowel wall from pressure by the bezoar, leading to perforation and peritonitis throughout the abdomen. In a variant of this condition, the so-called "Rapunzel syndrome", the bezoar can have a long tail extending down into the small bowel causing obstructive jaundice or pancreatitis. Bezoars can also cause protein-losing diarrhea, fatty diarrhea, or mechanical obstruction of the small bowel as well as the stomach. In some cases there have even been small bowel bezoars present along with the large one in the stomach.

Once having identified Ralph's problem, I tried to refer him to one of our local surgeons. However, having not had experience with this very rare disorder, the local surgeon recommended Ralph go to the university medical center for further characterization and removal of this mass, so my office made the arrangements for Ralph to be seen there. At the medical center the surgeons first performed an endoscopy which confirmed the presence of the bezoar and characterized it as a trichophytobezoar. This meant that in addition to hair from Ralph's mustache, there was a large amount of undigested food in the mass. They also found it was much too large to be fragmented and removed through the endoscope. The surgeons then recommended to Ralph that he have an open abdominal surgery, or laparotomy, for removal of the bezoar. In most cases laparotomy is considered the method of choice for removal of these lesions. At the time of his surgery, a three-pound bezoar was found and removed from his stomach. The surgeons then checked the remainder of his bowel and found no more bezoars.

Once this large mass was removed from his stomach, Ralph's symptoms rapidly resolved. Unfortunately, Ralph did not take the surgeon's advice to get rid of his mustache, nor did he stop chewing on it. As a result, his symptoms gradually returned. Within five years of his first surgery, Ralph had developed another trichobezoar, which required a second gastric surgery. Still, after the second surgery, Ralph did not shave his mustache. Though he has intermittent acid reflux, Ralph's upper GI x-rays since then have not found a third bezoar. Perhaps Ralph has finally stopped chewing on his mustache. In my thirty years of practice Ralph is the only patient I've ever seen with a trichobezoar, the human hair ball.

Heart Spells

Fannie was born and raised in the same eastern Kentucky county where she eventually met and married her husband, Tom, when she was just sixteen years old. Tom was a farmer in his twenties who had saved enough to buy his own farm, nestled between the hills they both loved so much. The land had an old farmhouse on it when they bought it, and within a few years Tom began adding on to the house as their six children came. Tom eventually developed the symptoms of heart disease but would not see a doctor about it. This eventually took him when Fannie was in her sixties. Sadly, she simply awoke one morning to find Tom lying next to her, unresponsive, having died silently during the night. After Tom's funeral Fannie continued to live on the farm alone. She never wanted to move from there if possible.

About ten years after Tom's death Fannie began having what she called "heart spells" during which she would "feel poorly". Her daughter took her to several doctors, none of whom ever found anything wrong with her heart. Several of the doctors said Fannie might be talking about heart problems to get attention, or perhaps she was becoming senile. Either way, no one believed she was having any kind of heart problem, neither her children nor the doctors.

Fannie was ninety-one years old when her youngest daughter, a well-to-do woman in a nearby large town, brought her to my office. She wanted me to examine her mother and prepare her for admission to a nursing home. According to the daughter, Fannie was demented. She would have periods where she was confused, and at such times she would just sit, staring off into space and not responding to those around her. Her daughter thought that this represented dementia. Her daughter was convinced that these so-called "heart spells" were a figment of Fannie's imagination, that her mother was now a hypochondriac and unable to take care herself at age ninety-one, and that she should not continue living alone.

As I began talking with Fannie, I could see right away that she was obviously not demented. She was alert, pleasant, and fully oriented to time, place, and circumstances. She was painfully aware that her daughter wanted her to go to a nursing home, something Fannie never wanted to do. Fannie said that she would be confused or not hear those who were talking to her only when she was having one of her "heart spells". In addition to feeling like her heart was racing, with a spell she would feel lightheaded, often be short of breath, and sometimes have trouble thinking clearly. She told me these spells would last up to half an hour as far she could tell, but most of the time they ended in just a few minutes. She didn't know if there was anything she did that caused them to start or stop. Other than the spells and the osteoarthritis of aging, Fannie was doing fairly well. She still did her own cooking, cleaning, housework, and grocery shopping. However, she would ask a neighbor to drive her to town for the grocery shopping or other errands, as she had become afraid to drive herself.

Fannie told me her daughter lived over an hour's drive from the farm in a large metropolitan area. She and her husband were quite well-to-do, but according to Fannie, she did not visit her very often. Fannie also told me she had never seen a doctor when she was having a "heart spell", as it would be over before anyone could get her to the doctor. She lived several minutes from the main road, and once there, it took another twenty minutes to get to the hospital, so I could readily understand why no one had seen her with the symptoms. She told me other doctors had done an EKG and an echocardiogram (an ultrasound of the heart), neither of which showed any abnormalities. Both had been done after the "heart spell" had ended.

As I began to examine the Fannie, she suddenly said, "Oh Doctor, I'm having one of those 'heart spells' right now." I quickly checked her pulse and found it was racing - very rapid but regular. I had an EKG machine in the office, and my nurse and I quickly connected Fannie to it. This was the first time Fannie had ever had an EKG done while she was having a spell, and her EKG showed an abnormal rapid heart rhythm known as supraventricular tachycardia.

The rhythm disturbance from which Fannie was suffering is associated with abnormal conduction within the heart's electrochemical conducting system. The conduction will start down a normal pathway and then back up an abnormal pathway to stimulate another heartbeat. This "circus movement" bypasses the normal pacemaker, leading to a heart rhythm which can be extremely fast. Fannie's heart rate was slightly over 150 beats per minute. It was remarkable that she had not suffered a heart attack from this fast a heart rate at her age.

Now that we at last had documentation that Fannie's "heart spells" were indeed due to a cardiac problem, she needed treatment to get her back to a normal rhythm right away. The first steps to try can be done at the bedside. First, we had Fannie take a deep breath and bear down as if to move her bowels. This increase in thoracic pressure, called a Valsalva maneuver, will often stimulate the vagus nerve, which will sometimes slow down the heart and convert it back to a normal rhythm. In her case, unfortunately, it did not work.

Next we attempted to stimulate the vagus nerve by massaging one of the specialized areas on the carotid artery called the carotid sinus. Before doing this it is essential to check both carotid pulses first so that one does not occlude with the pressure the patient's only functioning carotid artery! I quickly checked both of Fannie's carotid pulses, and both were full and strong. As I began massaging her left carotid sinus, the EKG machine, to which she was still connected, documented her conversion back to normal rhythm. Also, Fannie could tell immediately that this "heart spell" was over.

Had the carotid massage failed, we did have medication in the office that we could give intravenously to stop the abnormal rhythm. I was glad, though, that we did not have to use it. Interestingly, when I first began medical school, intravenous Digoxin, a digitalis preparation, was the drug of choice for this. By the time I finished my residency, intravenous verapamil, a calcium channel blocker, had become the drug of choice. Now intravenous adenosine is the preferred medication for converting this supraventricular rhythm back to a normal sinus rhythm.

Diagnosing the nature of Fannie's "heart spells" was very lucky. Fortunately, converting her out of this rhythm back into a normal one had been easy. Now came the hard part - explaining all this to her daughter. I called the daughter back into the examining room. I carefully explained to her that her mother was neither demented nor needing nursing home placement. I explained to her the reasons why I had come to those conclusions. I reviewed with her all the EKG tracings which documented that her mother was not a hypochondriac. I explained to her the nature of her mother's dysrhythmia, that it came in an unpredictable and paroxysmal fashion, and that it could not have been diagnosed by the cardiologist or any other doctor, had she not had the abnormal rhythm at the time the doctor examined her. Fannie's daughter was not happy at hearing this, but faced with the evidence of her mother's EKG tracings, she had no choice but to accept it. I prescribed a medication for Fannie to prevent these episodes, and the nurse arranged for her to return to the office in one month for recheck. She left with her daughter, and at least one of them was very pleased.

In a month Fannie returned, this time being driven by her neighbor. She reported she had had no further "heart spells" and that she felt wonderful on the medication. Fortunately, she also had had no side effects from the medication. Fannie continued to see me thereafter every three months and continued to do well for several more years. She was always grateful that I had proven her "heart spells" weren't "all in my head". Finally, at age ninety-seven she died in her sleep, as Tom had done, but for her it was from a stroke. She was found by her neighbor the next morning. She had gotten her wish to die in her own home and never go to a nursing home. I was glad for her.

Hernia

Ruby and her husband married in September of 1953 when they were just twenty years old. They had planned to have a large family, but over the years they were only able to have but two children, a son and a daughter. In their later years, however, they enjoyed many grandchildren. Her husband and she both worked intermittently, while she was also a homemaker and mother. Both of them became patients of mine when I first moved to Kansas. I would always enjoy chatting with them during their office visits as both of them had a great sense of humor. I saw him most often for emphysema, and her for management of adult-onset diabetes, hypertension, and high cholesterol.

Having been retired for several years and both being afflicted with osteoarthritis, the wear-and tear arthritis of aging, neither of them enjoyed the Kansas winter weather very much. They purchased a motor home and traveled to a small Texas town each autumn, returning each spring just as Texas was heating up. In Texas they would stay at the same motor home court each year, where they had developed long-time winter friends, "snow birds", who were doing the same thing they were to escape the winter's cold. Before their departure each November I would see them both to make sure all their prescriptions would last until their return. I also would have Ruby get her mammogram done each fall before their departure.

After several years of this routine, we found that the medications I had prescribed for Ruby for the osteoarthritis were no longer managing her arthritis pain. In addition some of her joints swelled and became reddened. I ordered blood tests on her, and unfortunately they were positive for crippling rheumatoid arthritis (RA). I referred her at once to a rheumatologist, an arthritis specialist, who assumed the management of the RA for her. He first started her on prednisone, a cortisone medication, to quiet it down, then began a series of infusions of what are called disease modifying drugs; these are medications which stop the progression of the arthritis and prevent crippling. Fortunately, these worked very well for her and led to a remission of the RA. However, this was not to be the end of her medical adventures.

About ten years ago, when Ruby was seventy years old, she decided she would finally have her cataract surgery that October before leaving for Texas. Prior to cataract surgery, the ophthalmologist would always consult the family doctor to evaluate the patient for safety of having this done under local anaesthesia. At this evaluation, I did a complete examination and found no reason for Ruby not to proceed with the surgery, and she did. At our visit that November she had fully recovered from the surgery and was pleased at how well she was seeing. We did her Pap smear and scheduled her for a mammogram. I was able to let her know these were normal before they took off for Texas.

During that winter in Texas, Ruby became more and more concerned that she was gaining weight. Her waist was enlarging so that her shorts and slacks no longer fit her. Her bathroom scales, however, showed very little weight gain. She could not understand how such a small change in her body weight could make such a big difference in how her clothes were fitting. She could not think of anything she had been doing differently in terms of activity or diet. Perhaps, she thought, she was eating more of the delicious south Texas food than she thought she was, so Ruby made an effort to reduce her portion sizes. This, however, seemed to make no difference. She decided she would discuss it with me upon their return to Kansas.

The weekend they drove back from Texas Ruby began having bad pain in her right groin. She went to the emergency room the day this started as it was too uncomfortable to ignore. She explained to the doctor how she had been gaining weight and how this pain had suddenly begun in her right groin. The doctor on duty at our local hospital ER checked her and told her she had a right inguinal (or groin) hernia. He prescribed some pain medication for her and advised her to wear a girdle until she could see a surgeon to fix the hernia. She did not understand why she should suddenly have a hernia, as she had not been lifting anything heavy or otherwise straining. Moreover, she was definitely not interested in wearing a girdle. She took the pain medication as prescribed by the

ER doctor and decided she would see me the next week about this before going to a surgeon.

The following Monday she came to my office to see what could be done for her groin pain. On examining Ruby I found she had a basketball-sized lesion in the pelvis extending up to the size of a twenty-week pregnancy. (This would correspond to a mass extending about two inches above her navel.) A pelvic exam performed at that time confirmed that it was likely an ovarian mass. This was a dramatic change from her examination the previous fall for her cataract surgery.

Groin pain such as Ruby was experiencing could indeed suggest a hernia in men or boys. However, due to their different anatomy, such inguinal hernias were rather rare among women and girls. When a woman might experience such pain is in middle to late pregnancy when the round ligament of the uterus is stretched by the growing baby. This ligament extends down into the groin where it ends within the inguinal connective tissues. In Ruby's case her right round ligament was being stretched by a massive right ovarian tumor.

That day I obtained an ultrasound of Ruby's pelvis which showed a large part-cystic and part-solid mass. We then scheduled Ruby for a CAT scan of abdomen and pelvis with and without contrast. This scan would enable us not only to characterize better the mass seen on ultrasound but also let us know if there were any evidence of metastatic spread of this likely cancerous tumor. Unfortunately, in addition to the cystic and solid complex mass seen in the pelvis, the CAT scan also identified an enlargement of her left adrenal gland that might represent possible metastatic disease. I shared this information with her and her husband and immediately referred her to a gynecologist.

Approximately a week later the gynecologist took her to the operating room for removal of this lesion. I was able to assist with that surgery. Although the gynecologist was a very careful and skillful surgeon, it was not possible to excise the basketball-sized cyst and the solid portions of the mass without rupturing the cyst with some of the fluid leaking into the abdomen. This fluid likely contained cancer cells, so this leakage increased the chances of cancer spread. When it was finally removed, this tumor filled one of the old stainless steel basins that were once used for hospital bed baths.

On pathologic exam Ruby's tumor was diagnosed as cystadenocarcinoma of the ovary, a cystic form of ovarian cancer. Unfortunately, one month after her surgery, another CAT scan of the abdomen showed a new small lesion in the liver. The lesion in the adrenal gland at that point was unchanged and was felt to be benign. Approximately two weeks later Ruby had her first visit with the oncologist, a cancer specialist. She was then started on chemotherapy for the ovarian cancer, which cause some nausea and the loss of her hair. Other than this, Ruby tolerated the chemotherapy quite well.

It has now been ten years since Ruby's surgery. She has since been widowed, but fortunately she has shown no evidence of recurrence of the ovarian cancer. I spoke last month with her granddaughter, who reports Ruby is still very active and enjoying life. She has been able to keep her diabetes under good control, and the rheumatologist has kept her rheumatoid arthritis in remission. In retrospect I am really glad that Ruby came to me right away about her "hernia". To this day I cannot understand how the emergency room doctor could miss a mass so large that it looked like a seventy-year-old woman was twenty weeks pregnant!

HIV Test

For two of my thirty years of medicine I was employed by the federal government in a nine-to-five position. It was for me an important time in my life not to be working so many hours or taking after-hours call. My two younger sons were playing high school football during those years, and with this position I was able to attend many of their games. I was very happy to have had the opportunity to watch my sons play football and cheer for them. However, working for the federal government came with a substantial cut in income. In order to continue to earn enough to pay my older son's way through college, I did moonlighting work in the emergency room of a small-town hospital nearby. It was at that hospital that I had one of the strangest patient encounters I've ever experienced.

Steve had certainly not had an easy life. He grew up poor and while in high school became involved in the illegal drug trade. After high school, he continued selling illegal drugs until he was finally arrested, prosecuted, convicted, and sent to state prison. Steve was a fairly short, thin man with an unruly crop of strawberry blonde hair. Given his small stature, he probably did not have pleasant experiences with other inmates while incarcerated. He was fortunate to be let out on parole after serving only five years.

Apparently the very day of his parole, Steve had hitchhiked a ride into the small town where I was working in the emergency room. However, in addition to the ride, he tried to rob the driver and his front-seat passenger at knife-point. Just then the driver saw a state trooper vehicle proceeding toward him. He changed lanes, driving right at the oncoming officer, and then stopped. The state trooper, Adam, had been an officer for over fifteen years, and this was the first time someone had deliberately done this to him. He stopped his cruiser, turned on his emergency lights, and approached the other car. That was when things got crazy.

As Adam walked toward the vehicle, stopped directly in front of his own, both the driver and front-seat passenger jumped out their respective doors with their hands in the air, shouting that the man in the back seat, Steve, was a hitchhiker trying to rob them. Adam then had those two step away from their vehicle. He opened the back door and ordered Steve to drop his knife, then step out of the car. Steve began swearing, yelling obscenities, and calling Adam the "n" word. He tried to stab Adam repeatedly while refusing to exit the car. Eventually Adam was able to grab Steve just above an ankle and drag him out of the vehicle. A struggle ensued in which Steve bit Adam twice on the arm, repeatedly trying to stab him and get away. Adam had to hit Steve on the head three times during the altercation to subdue him. He finally got Steve's knife away from him, wrestled him to the ground, and put him in handcuffs. Adam then escorted Steve to his cruiser, radioed in his identity, and learned that Steve had been paroled that very day. Then, since both of them had injuries, Adam drove to the emergency room where I would see them both. Adam was followed by two officers from the local police department who would watch over Steve while Adam would be treated in a separate room.

Steve had been bleeding from the scalp since being struck with Adam's baton. He had three small lacerations on his scalp where he had been hit with it. He had some red marks on his arms where he apparently tried to block Adam's blows, and there was a little "road rash" or abrasion in a few areas from the altercation. While I was examining him to find the extent of his injuries, Steve was flanked by the two local police officers. He was yelling as loud as he could in a sing-song voice about Adam and his race in general, and about how he would revenge himself on Adam. He did quiet down a little when I asked him if he had any other injuries and responded, "No, but I'm going to kill that n***** cop!", and resumed his yelling.

I asked the nurse to cleanse Steve's lesser wounds while I repaired the lacerations to his scalp. With the two policemen standing on each side of him he agreed to hold still while I was working, but he continued screaming racial epithets hoping that Adam in the next room would hear him. Once his scalp lacerations were repaired and his lesser wounds dressed, I again asked Steve if he had any other injuries. Again he replied that he did not, immediately resuming his yelling. Since he did not know when his last tetanus shot was, I had the nurse give him one as I left to attend Adam. Walking into the second room where Adam was waiting for me, I could hear clearly all the things Steve was yelling, so I knew Adam had been hearing all that as well.

About three times Steve's size and an experienced officer, Adam did not have any injuries other than the two bite marks on his forearm where Steve bit him during their altercation. Both of the bites had broken the skin. I asked the nurse to cleanse both areas and apply sterile dressings. Since human bites are among the most contaminated of all wounds, I prescribed Adam a broad-spectrum antibiotic. While I was completing his prescription and emergency room record, Adam asked me if I could obtain an HIV test on Steve since he had just been released from prison. Given Steve's size and appearance, it was not unlikely that he might have acquired this through sexual assault while incarcerated.   I told Adam that I could not test Steve without his consent, but I would try.   I completed the paperwork for Adam and returned to the other room, wondering how I could obtain consent from someone so out of control and angry with the arresting officer. Then the solution hit me - reverse the concerns about HIV.

Steve was still shouting racial slurs when I pointed out to him that in biting Adam he had gotten some of Adam's blood into his mouth.   I informed Steve that it was not likely that he had acquired HIV with that exchange of body fluids, but one could never tell. I asked if he would like to be tested for HIV to establish his baseline status. He said he definitely wanted the test and would sign the consent form for it. We then had Steve sign the written consent for HIV testing, and the lab drew his blood for the test. He never seemed to suspect that we were drawing the blood more for the benefit of Adam than for him. Steve was then escorted to the local jail, where he would be housed until he was sent back to prison for the violation of his parole.

About three months later, I received a telephone call from the hospital's attorney regarding the care I had provided for Steve. The attorney was concerned that I had not documented a rectal exam on Steve, who was now claiming that Adam had taken him out to the edge of town, sexually assaulted him, and then brought him to the hospital. I advised the attorney that if he had a cut on the top of his head, he would not likely accept having a rectal examination done; it was certainly not medically necessary. Moreover, I informed the attorney that Steve twice denied any other injuries at the time he was in the emergency room, and this was documented in the ER record. That conversation with the attorney for the hospital was the last I heard about Steve. Apparently, the threatened lawsuit against the hospital and me never materialized. I still consider this to be one of the most bizarre experiences I have had in the practice of medicine. Fortunately, for both Adam and Steve, the HIV test was negative.

HMO

In the 1980s there was an explosion of new technologies and medications. The CAT scanner was becoming more and more widely used. This machine could solve diagnostic riddles that used to take weeks and multiple, sometimes invasive, tests to resolve. As a neurologist friend put it, "One CT scan is worth ten neurologists!" when it came to brain pathology. Also, the MRI was just coming into its own as another amazing diagnostic tool. However, all these technologic advances as well as all the new medications were not inexpensive. Like flat-screen televisions or any other breakthrough, there was tremendous cost involved in the research and development that produced such wonders.

As these technologic and pharmacologic marvels emerged, insurance companies resisted having to pay for them. Though the cost of government and college education had risen even faster, they raised a big outcry against the increases in medical costs. Insurance companies then developed new ways of controlling their costs, one of which was to shift cost risk to the physician. The new product, called a "health maintenance organization" or HMO for short, would pay the doctor a set monthly "capitation" fee from which the doctor had to pay for all the medical care for the patients in his or her panel.

The insurance companies thought this would pressure the doctor to order fewer and other - but most importantly, cheaper - testing and treatments even though most physicians were already doing that where appropriate. The HMO doctor could even be paid a bonus if the costs at the end of the year were less than projected. This created a perverse incentive to do less than the best for the patient. To me this was not a system in which I wanted to be involved. I have always tried to keep expenses down for my patients, since they have to pay a portion of the costs, but without the pressure to do less for them. In 1990 when practicing in Michigan, I saw first-hand the kind of problems that an HMO-style system would generate.

On a Saturday in June of that year I was working in the emergency room of our local hospital. Barely ten miles away was a very popular Midwestern campground with two large lakes, multiple recreation areas, and several miles of gravel paths around the lakes and connecting many areas of the complex. Early that afternoon a young man, Jonathan, was brought to us from that campground by his mother. They were from nearby Kalamazoo and vacationing there that summer. Having had a terrible bicycle accident, Jonathan was in horrific pain.

Apparently after lunch Jonathan and his brother, Peter, decided to have a bicycle race around the lakes and through the activity areas. Halfway through their race Jonathan went around a corner much too fast on the gravel pathway, and his bike slid out from under him. Wearing only a tank top, shorts, and tennis shoes with no socks, Jonathan slid approximately twenty-five yards, deeply imbedding gravel, dirt, mud, and grass into almost twenty-five percent of his entire skin. Peter stopped immediately and helped his brother make his way slowly back to where their family was camping. His mother brought Jonathan to us immediately.

Jonathan was in horrific pain. The young man was thirteen years old but quite big for his age, almost six feet tall and weighing nearly two hundred pounds. His tank top was shredded on the right side as were his shorts. His right shoe was gone. On examination he was found to have extensive "road rash" involving the right side of his face, right upper arm, right elbow and wrist, and right hip and leg all the way down to his ankle. Deeply embedded into the skin of these areas were dirt, mud, grass, and gravel. The entire area was oozing blood and clear lymph. Again, the area of his injury represented approximately twenty-five percent of his total body surface. Jonathan had no other significant injuries, but his whole body was shaking from the intense pain. It was immediately obvious to the nurse and me that cleansing and debridement (picking out all the foreign material and badly damaged tissue) would not be a simple task. With the debris so deeply embedded, failure to remove it could lead to severe infection as well as permanent tattooing of his skin.

I spoke with Jonathan's mother and advised her I would call in one of our local surgeons to take her son to the operating room so these wounds could be scrubbed, debrided, and then properly dressed under light general anesthesia without causing him even more extreme pain. I advised her I did not feel it appropriate to do this without anesthesia. She agreed to this approach to treatment, but as I started to call the surgeon, she told me that they belonged to an HMO in Kalamazoo. I would have to call their HMO physician for prior authorization before proceeding. I quickly hung up the telephone. She gave me the telephone number of the HMO doctor, whom I then called.

I explained to the on-call HMO doctor the nature of Jonathan's injuries, stressing how extensive they were. I told him it would take vigorous scrubbing to cleanse the wounds properly. Nonetheless, the HMO doctor on-call refused to authorize our taking him to the OR for general anesthesia. He suggested I just apply lidocaine jelly (a topical anaesthetic) to the wounds then scrub them in the emergency room. He said if I was unwilling to proceed that way, I was to have his mother bring Jonathan to his office in Kalamazoo where he would do it there. Again I stressed to this doctor the depth of injury as well as the extensive nature of the "road rash". Still he refused to authorize taking him to the OR for this.

When I informed his mother that the HMO doctor on call refused to authorize payment for the care I had recommended for Jonathan, she became extremely and vocally angry. She told me that as soon as their vacation was over, this would no longer be their insurance. She had thought to save money by signing up for the HMO, and indeed, they did have a somewhat lower premium. However, they were now facing a much lower standard of care. She insisted on driving Jonathan to the office of the on-call HMO doctor. The nurse and I applied sterile wet-to-dry saline dressings to the injured areas. I had the nurse give Jonathan a shot for pain. His mother then loaded him into their car and drove him to Kalamazoo. I asked before she left to please let me know how this turned out, and I gave her my card.

Two weeks later Jonathan's mother called me from Kalamazoo. She had gone to the doctor's office and demanded that he permit the care which we had recommended. Under mother's threats to sue and, especially, to call to the doctor's office a camera crew from the local TV station (where she just happened to be a newscaster), he relented and authorized Jonathan to have the care I had recommended. His mother told me her son had recovered and had no scars or tattooing marks on his face, arm, or leg from the bike accident. She thanked me again for having taken care of Jonathan and told me they were no longer HMO members.

This was just one of many such cases that highlighted for me the deficiencies of healthcare delivery systems which focus primarily on controlling costs instead of serving the patient. I had always been doubtful of the wisdom of such an arrangement. After seeing what almost happened to Jonathan that day, I decided I would never involve myself professionally with any HMO or similar system. I have thus remained free to use my best judgment for the most appropriate and cost-effective care for each patient without pressure from a third party. However, in this regard, with our recent federal laws, I fear for the future of medicine.

Intussusception

It was 3 a.m. when Mrs. Jones called me, extremely distraught about her son Marcus, a cute tow-headed green-eyed boy not yet two years old. An experienced mother of four, she told me Marcus had eaten a good supper, played happily after dinner showing no signs of illness, and had gone to bed apparently feeling fine. However, for the last two hours Marcus would scream out in pain about every five to ten minutes, seeming to strain to move his bowels, then falling back asleep as the pain seemed to subside. She reported that in the last hour he also had two episodes of vomiting. She told me he had not had any fever, chills, or other systemic signs of illness or toxicity. Mrs. Jones told me that she had never seen this kind of thing with any of her children. Suspecting intussusception, I told her to take Marcus to the emergency room immediately, and I would meet them there. I then quickly dressed and drove to the hospital where I awaited their arrival.

Intussusception is a disease of small children, usually occurring between three months and two years of age. No one really knows why this happens, or why it happens four times more often in boys than in girls. In rare cases an anatomic structural abnormality, such as a tumor, may be found to be the cause in this age group. Intussusception is the bowel telescoping in on itself. Most of the time it is the end of the ileum, the last part of the small intestine, that telescopes into the first part of the colon. Rarely the appendix will form the advancing apex of an intussusception. As the more proximal portion of the bowel telescopes in, it will pull in its blood vessels as well. When the outer layer of this "telescope" then cramps down on the inner one, it can cut off blood supply to the inner portion, resulting in swelling, pain, and even gangrenous death of the intestine if this condition goes on too long.

Blood-tinged stools may be passed in intussusception, and up to two-thirds of affected children will pass a stool with dark red blood and mucus, the so-called "currant jelly" stool. Most of these children do not have a significant fever early on and indeed will seem well between the paroxysms of pain. This is a true medical emergency as intestinal gangrene, shock, and even death can occur if this is not diagnosed and treated promptly. Fortunately, the colicky symptoms are usually too classic to be missed. Occasionally, though, a child will not seem to have much pain, and the diagnosis might be overlooked at first. Marcus's case, fortunately, was rather typical.

When Marcus and his mother arrived at the emergency room, I examined him and found his abdomen to be slightly tender, flat, and with an ill-defined sausage-shaped mass in the right upper quadrant. When he had an episode of pain, the mass was even more prominent. I next performed a gentle rectal exam and, fortunately, found there was no blood yet in his stool. We next obtained a plain abdominal x-ray which showed an abnormal density in the area of the suspected intussusception. At this point we called in the radiologist on duty.

The best early treatment for intussusception is emergency reduction of the telescoping bowel with either an air or barium enema. When this procedure is unsuccessful, or if the intussusception is too long-standing, surgical reduction is necessary. Moreover, in cases where there is an anatomic structural abnormality causing the intussusception, an enema reduction is rarely successful. In cases of fairly short duration, such as Marcus', when there are no signs of bowel perforation, the air or barium pressure under fluoroscopic guidance by the radiologist will often reduce the intussusception and relieve the bowel obstruction it caused. Some radiologists prefer to use air as it is felt to be less likely to cause perforation than barium. Others, however, prefer barium as it provides better pressure and is felt more likely to be successful in reducing the intussusception.

As soon as the radiologist arrived in the hospital, a scout film was obtained and a Foley catheter placed in Marcus' rectum. His buttocks were taped together, he was turned on his back, and the barium solution was then allowed to flow in by gravity. The radiologist made a special effort to make sure that no one would press or even touch Marcus' abdomen during the procedure. With the fluoroscope we were able to see the column of barium filling the distal colon quickly, then slowly reaching the site where the intussusception had occurred. In Marcus's case it was at

107

the junction of the colon and the ileum, the terminal end of the small intestine.

Once the barium column reached this spot, within moments there was sudden free filling of the distal small bowel with barium. With this Marcus' symptoms were immediately and completely relieved. Upon removal of the tape and catheter he at once passed much of the barium. He walked on his own from the x-ray department back to the emergency room with a big smile on his face, carrying the teddy bear the hospital always gave to little patients such as Marcus.

I explained to Mrs. Jones how well the barium enema had worked, and she could see how much better Marcus was. I advised her regarding the risk of recurrence, about ten percent in these cases, and asked her to call me later that morning to report on his status. Fortunately, Marcus had no recurrence, and later that day Mrs. Jones reported he was doing fine. I was glad she had called me right away so that we could save Marcus from surgery for the intussusception, a true pediatric emergency.

Itchy

It was early on a Thursday morning, as I was preparing to see the first patient of the day, when Sam walked in wanting an appointment. He said, "I've been itching all over, and nothing seems to help. Also, my urine has been getting dark." I replied, "Sam, you just earned yourself a blood test out at the hospital this morning." He replied, "But Doc! I'm not fasting." "It doesn't matter," I said, "you're getting it now anyway. You need it this very morning."

I had first met Sam when I joined the Knights of Columbus after moving to Parsons. We had worked together on several Knights projects and became friends as well as doctor and patient. Back then Sam worked for a major national firm in which he had worked his way up to regional supervisor. Now he was "retired" from that and working for a local company. When our parish had a pilgrimage trip to Poland, we couldn't go, but our wives roomed together on the trip and grew to be good friends, too. So Sam and I had a history with each other outside of medicine.

Most folks with generalized itching suspect they have some type of an allergy, either to something new to which they have been exposed, or to a pollen or other environmental allergen. Most of the time, however, such an allergic reaction develops from something to which the person had been exposed many times in the past. In Sam's case not only did he have generalized itching, but his urine was dark as well. This combination of symptoms suggested obstruction of his bile duct. The bile ducts are like a tree whose main branches, the right and left hepatic duct emerge from their respective lobes of the liver. These two then join to form the common bile duct not far "upstream" from the gall bladder. This common duct then runs from above the gallbladder, around to the pancreas, and empties alongside the pancreatic duct into the duodenum, the first part of the small intestine. When the bile duct is obstructed, bile salts build up in the skin causing itching. Moreover, with duct obstruction the bile is then excreted in the urine, darkening it. Since the bile, which gives stool its brown color, cannot be excreted in the intestine, the obstruction can eventually lead to having white stools. At Sam's age there was a significant chance that he might have cancer of the pancreas blocking the common bile duct. Sam had had a previous cholecystectomy, the removal of the gallbladder, so gall stones blocking the duct seemed less likely, though this can still occur even after removal of the gallbladder.

Just after noon that day I received the report on Sam's blood test. As I had suspected, it showed an elevated bilirubin and elevated liver enzymes. This confirmed my suspicion of bile duct blockage and explained the itch and the dark urine. Now we had to find out what was causing it. I called Sam at work right away and informed him of the result and what it meant. I told him, "Now you have earned yourself a CAT scan of the abdomen this afternoon." He replied, "I'm still not fasting, and I'm busy at work. Can we schedule it for next week?" I responded, "You're done working for the day. We need the CAT scan now." Sam replied, "What's the big rush?" "Sam," I said, " one of the most common causes of bile duct obstruction in your age group is cancer of the pancreas." He immediately agreed to go for the scan that afternoon and would bring Terri, his wife, with him. I told him I would meet them at the hospital right after the scan was done and let them know the results.

I met Sam and Terri in the x-ray waiting room just after having reviewed the CAT scan with the radiologist. Fortunately we were alone in the room. I told them there was no tumor visible on the scan, but Sam's common bile duct was about the size of my thumb. A normal common bile duct would be about the size of a fat ball-point refill. Although tumor could not be seen on the CAT scan, it was still possible to have a small cancer right at the outlet, blocking the drainage of both the bile and pancreatic ducts. I informed them of this and that our next step would be an ERCP, the endoscopic retrograde cannulation of the pancreas. This test, done by a gastroenterologist, involves general anaesthesia with the passage of a scope through the stomach, to the duodenum, and directly into the bile duct or pancreatic duct. This test would give us the final diagnosis, or so I thought. Sam agreed to proceed with this.

While we were sitting there in the x-ray waiting room, I called a trusted gastroenterologist in Joplin and explained to him the situation. Understanding the urgency of the situation and thus the need for a rapid diagnosis, he agreed to see Sam at 4:00 PM the next day and do the ERCP then. Sam agreed. That Friday Sam had the ERCP test in Joplin.

On Monday Terri stopped by the office to update me. There had been a dozen deep-green gallstones in Sam's bile duct. She said they looked like little sweet pickles, each almost an inch long. No wonder his duct was blocked! Once these were removed, the duct was able to drain. However, the outlet was at risk of swelling shut with all these stones being removed through it, so a stent had to be placed to keep the duct draining until the swelling went down. Sam was to go back in two weeks to have the stent removed. Terri told me he was feeling much better, and his urine was no longer dark. Unfortunately, it would take several more days for the itching to subside.

Two weeks later Sam went back to Joplin to have the stent removed. At that time the gastroenterologist injected some contrast dye up into the bile duct tree to make sure there were no further stones. The right hepatic duct would not fill with contrast, suggesting the possibility of a retained stone. He elected to leave the stent in place for another two weeks. Two weeks later Sam had the test again. Once again the right hepatic duct would not fill with contrast. This time the gastroenterologist passed an instrument up into the right hepatic duct to investigate. There was no stone. Instead he found a solid mass in the duct, which he biopsied.

Sam and Terri were quietly anxious for a few days, awaiting the results of the biopsy. It showed cholangiocarcinoma, an aggressive cancer of bile ducts. Most often this is a fatal diagnosis. These cancers tend to remain quiet, not causing any symptoms, until they are widespread and incurable. Other times such cancers will be very small at discovery and yet still be incurable.

The gastroenterologist made arrangements for Sam to be seen at a major medical center in St. Louis, Missouri. There he underwent removal of the right hepatic duct as well as part of the right lobe of the liver. The surgeons took enough tissue to ensure, as best they could, that the margins of the remaining tissues would be free from cancer. Next they cut loose a piece of small bowel, joining the remaining bowel ends together. With the piece of small intestine thus freed up, they created a new right hepatic duct for what remained of the right lobe of the liver. It appeared that they had gotten all of the cancer, and Sam was sent to the recovery room. Through his stay in St. Louis Sam lost weight and became rather weak. Once home he gradually began walking again. At first he walked just two houses down the street and back. As the weeks went by, he regained his strength and appetite and was able to walk more.

Six weeks after surgery Sam and Terri returned to St. Louis where another CAT scan was performed. Unfortunately, the doctors in St. Louis thought they saw a recurrence of the tumor at the site of the surgery. He was then sent back here for a consultation with the oncologist, a cancer specialist, to see what could be done for him. The oncologist here discussed the situation with them and ordered a PET scan, short for Positron Emission Tomography. This test would confirm if there was any remaining tumor from the cholangiocarcinoma. The PET scan is much more sensitive than a CAT scan or even an MRI for detecting the spread of most cancers, including cholangiocarcinoma.

The PET scan showed no evidence of any tumor. Apparently what was seen on the CAT scan in St. Louis was just post-surgical scarring and not new cancer. Sam, indeed, had had a surgical cure from a usually fatal cancer. To this day he has done well. Thanks to itching and a dozen gallstones, Sam was spared an early death.

Kentucky Football

In my third and final year of family medicine residency I had some elective time available to me. As the father of an athletic daughter and three sons, I knew our children were likely to be active in high school sports; the two older ones were already involved with elementary school and city league sports. One of the second-year residents apparently "knew someone who knew someone" and was given a chance to learn sports medicine under the tutelage of the athletic trainer for the Kentucky's famous basketball team. However, I felt that I would have greater opportunity for learning by working with Kentucky's not-so- well-known football team. I discussed this with my faculty adviser who asked me bluntly how I thought that working with the football team was an educational opportunity. I explained to him that I was going to be practicing medicine in a small town where I would be treating high school athletic injuries on a regular basis. With this in mind, he conceded that this would be an educational rotation, and he would approve it, provided the head athletic trainer for football, Mr. Al Green, was also amenable to the idea.

This was a time of turnover for Kentucky football. Though he had been head football coach at Virginia Tech and Maryland, this would be the first year that the former Kentucky player, Coach Jerry Claiborne, would be back coaching at his alma mater. As is always the case with head coaching changes, there was a lot of activity in the football program adjusting to the new coach and his style of work. Assistant coaches and other personnel were unsure of their jobs at first, and it was during this time of uncertainty that I had to approach Al Green, the head football trainer, with the idea of a family medicine resident working under his direction to learn that aspect of sports medicine. As I explained to Mr. Green, I knew quite well how to manage strains, sprains, and other sports injuries in the clinic setting, but I knew nothing about how they were handled on the sideline or in the training room. Al then asked me if I planned to come there to tell them how to do their jobs. I advised him that would not be the case at all; I was coming there to learn under his direction what I didn't know, not to show off what I knew already. He looked me in the eye and said warily, "Okay, we'll see how it goes."

That year, 1982, was a tough one for Kentucky football. As is so often the case with a change in head coach, there had been some turnover of player personnel as well. That season the Kentucky football program had a final record of 0-10-1. Back then games could still end in a tie. Two years later, however, Jerry Claiborne led Kentucky to 9-3 record, and Kentucky won the Hall of Fame bowl, finishing the season ranked 19th nationally. As bad as the 1982 season was for the team, for me it was a great opportunity to learn. As I found out very quickly, the losing team generally tends to have more injuries -and more severe ones - than the winning team. I thus had the opportunity to learn sideline and training room management of a variety of sports injuries. Of course, the more severe injuries would be referred to the team doctors, well-known local orthopedic surgeons, but as a family physician I still had the chance to learn how top-notch orthopedists handled such cases. I was also able to observe the recovery and rehabilitation process, and how these were assessed by expert athletic trainers. In later years, when I was practicing in small towns with no athletic trainer, this experience proved to be a great help.

Interestingly, since most of the Kentucky football games were broadcast on a delayed basis at night, my children would stay up late those Saturday nights to see if they could spot their father on television. Twice they did so, though the first time was rather embarrassing for me. One of the first things Al Green had told me - and repeatedly - was that when standing on the sideline during a football game, you should never turn your back to the field. Unfortunately, at one point during the Kentucky-Georgia football game, I was asked a question and turned my head to answer. At that instant I felt someone grab my coat collar and jerk me backward off my feet. It was Al Green. He had pulled me aside seconds before Herschel Walker, Georgia's outstanding All-American running back, ran out of bounds right where I had been standing. It was a lesson I never forgot. Herschel Walker rushed thirty-four times that game for a hundred fifty-two yards, a game which Georgia won 27-14. Herschel Walker went on to win the Heisman Trophy that year, and Georgia was voted the national champion of college football for the 1982 season. Back then they voted on such things.

The children's second opportunity to see me on television occurred when the trainers, including me, ran onto the field for a Kentucky player whose shoulder was dislocated. Al quickly diagnosed the problem and motioned for the orthopedist and the motorized cart. The game was stopped while the cart came out on the field. We helped the injured player onto the cart and rode with him back to the locker room. Once there, the orthopedist injected the shoulder with a local anesthetic and reduced the dislocation. Though that player was unable to return to the field for that game, I was later able to watch his rehabilitation from the injury. This was the first time I had had that opportunity, though it was the third time I had witnessed a dislocated shoulder reduction. Watching me on the television replay that night, my youngest son said to his mother, "Now Daddy's a real doctor!" Apparently he had not been impressed that I was licensed after the completion of my internship over a year prior, or that I would become board certified in a matter of months. No, it was being on television that made me a "real doctor" in his eyes!

One of the things that Al Green taught me personally was how to tape an ankle quickly. With eighty-five football players (a hundred seventy ankles) to tape before practices, there was no time to fool around. He showed me how to apply the underwrap and then begin the taping process. While he could tape an ankle within seconds, it took me a lot longer. Perhaps because of that, one of the freshman players, a wide receiver, always seemed to seek me out to tape his ankles. He was a most pleasant young man with a great sense of humor, always polite and patient with my slow taping. As I gradually improved, he was quite complementary to me. I never forgot the name of that wide receiver, Joker Phillips, who later went on to play professionally and eventually become the head coach of the football program at the University of Kentucky.

I was very glad to have had the opportunity to work with Al Green, Coach Claiborne, and the other staff and players on the Kentucky football team that year. I learned a tremendous amount from that experience which stood me in good stead when working as a small-town doctor taking care of athletic injuries. For his part Mr. Green was quite pleased with how well my six-week rotation with Kentucky football had gone. Since then the sports medicine rotation with the football team has become a very popular option with the family medicine program. I am proud of having helped to build the relationship between the two programs, and I hope that the opportunity continues to be an elective rotation available to other family medicine residents.

Leukemia

When I first moved to Parsons in 1994, there were no full-time ER doctors covering that department around the clock. We family physicians were assigned to a call schedule, in which we took turns covering the ER. It may not have been an ideal system, but it was the best we could do in our small community. It wasn't until several years later that we were able to attract and keep full-time emergency doctors on staff. It was in September 1995, while I was on call for the ER, that I first met Paul.

Paul was a well-known businessman in town and was always very busy. He would rarely take time off to see a doctor if he could avoid it. However, on this particular occasion, he had no choice. He had awoken in the middle of the night vomiting bright red blood and having dark bloody diarrhea. Paul reported to me in the ER that he was very weak, dizzy, lightheaded, and felt like his heart was racing. Paul denied having had heartburn, indigestion, or abdominal pain. At fifty years of age he had been relatively healthy until this occurred. He did not use tobacco, very rarely used alcohol, and did not take in much caffeine. All three of those substances increase stomach acid output and can contribute to the development of ulcers, and a bleeding ulcer was the most likely explanation for his symptoms.

On examination I found Paul to be very pale, cool, and sweaty. His heart was indeed racing, suggesting he had lost much more blood than he realized. The almost-black stool found on his rectal exam was strongly positive for blood. His initial blood count in the ER showed a hemoglobin of only 7.0, the normal hemoglobin for a man his age being 14.0 to 18.0. A low hemoglobin is the hallmark of anemia, and his was profound. Paul's extremely low hemoglobin confirmed that he had had a major blood loss, and it certainly explained why his heart was racing. There was no question of his being able to go back home. As a busy businessman, he did not want to be hospitalized; as ill as he was, he had no other option.

In the hospital I had to transfuse Paul with four units of blood before I could get his hemoglobin up to 10.

From a hemoglobin of 10, most patients with healthy bone marrow could make enough blood to get them back to the normal range. In addition, most patients could function rather well without dizziness or lightheadedness once their hemoglobin was back to 10. Suspecting a bleeding ulcer, I also began Paul on medication for this and consulted one of our local surgeons to see him. The surgeon performed an upper gastrointestinal endoscopy and found that Paul indeed had a bleeding peptic ulcer. Fortunately, the biopsy the surgeon did at the time of the endoscopy showed no cancer. Within three days Paul felt much better and was able to be discharged home on medication for ulcer as well as iron replacement. Arrangements were made for him to see me in the office in follow-up four weeks after discharge for further care. The four weeks would give his bone marrow time to build his blood count back up. ·

When I saw him in the office after those four weeks, Paul looked much better than he did at the time of discharge. He had good color in his face again and walked with much more energy. Once again, on his office examination, he had no epigastric (upper stomach) tenderness at all. He had not vomited any further blood, though he was still passing some black stools, this time because of the iron pills he was taking rather than from bleeding. I was pleased that Paul was feeling so much better and looking so much better, but I was concerned that his first symptom of having an ulcer was the vomiting of a large amount of blood. Surely there was some way we could monitor him to try to catch recurrent peptic ulcer disease as early as possible so he could be spared another hospitalization with such severe illness and so much blood loss.

I talked with Paul about ways we could monitor him. Perhaps the least expensive would be to check his stool every month for occult blood. This test would find even microscopic amounts of blood in the stool.

Peptic ulcers begin oozing small amounts of blood long before they bleed enough to cause vomiting of

blood. If we could detect that early bleeding, we could save him from another hospitalization. Paul, however, did not want anything to do with checking monthly stool specimens. He shook his head saying, "There is no way I am going to fool with that. Isn't there some other way?"

I suggested that we could do a monthly CBC, complete blood count, which would tell us if his hemoglobin was dropping from slow chronic blood loss. However, his insurance company would likely not pay for that since it is not a usual or normal way to treat ulcer disease. Nonetheless, I thought this might be appropriate in his case. Paul then asked me, "How much would that cost if I wanted to pay for it myself?" I checked with the clinic lab and found this would cost him $12 a month. Paul immediately decided that he would prefer to pay for that himself rather than collect a stool specimen each month and carry it to the clinic lab for testing for occult blood.

For nearly a full year we did the monthly blood counts on Paul, always checking carefully to make sure that there was no drop in his hemoglobin. The CBCs initially showed gradual improvement in his hemoglobin level and then remained in the normal range. He was pleased with this method of monitoring and reported he had not had any more black stools. However, after about a year of monitoring, he had an abnormal blood test. This time, however, from one month to the next, his white blood cell count went from the normal range of 5,000 to 10,000 up to 44,000 with many immature types of cells. In addition, his platelet count - the tiny bits of cells that form blood clots -

went from the normal (100,000 to 300,000) to over 500,000.

As soon as I received this report, I immediately called Paul to ask how he was feeling, as a severe infection might do this. He told me he felt well except for some unexplained fatigue. Clearly I could not blame the white blood cell count on an infection, since he had no signs or symptoms of infection and certainly no fever. He thought perhaps the fatigue might be from his hemoglobin having slipped down a little bit. Unfortunately, that was not the case. I asked him to come back to the clinic right away for a repeat blood count. He did so, and the results were the same. They suggested leukemia. We made arrangements for a bone marrow examination the next day; this confirmed that Paul had suddenly developed chronic myelogenous leukemia.

Like almost half of the patients diagnosed with this leukemia, Paul was almost without symptoms, and the disease was found simply because we were doing the monthly blood tests to monitor his peptic ulcer disease. Most patients who develop this leukemia complain of fatigue, weight loss, and generally feeling bad. Rarely, they will present with clots from a high platelet count, or bleeding due to a low platelet count. The average age for diagnosis is fifty to fifty-five years, and Paul fell into that range. In the vast majority of cases there is no external agent, such as a chemical or radiation, incriminated in the development of this leukemia. Genetic examination of his bone marrow confirmed the presence of what is known as the Philadelphia chromosome; it is seen only in this type of leukemia.

Once I explained the bone marrow findings to him, Paul and his wife, Laura, decided he would go to a nearby major cancer medical center for treatment. There he was initially begun on interferon and a drug called Ara-C. This treatment, which he took for almost five years, led to dramatic reduction of the presence of the Philadelphia chromosome in his bone marrow. Unfortunately, it also caused significant toxicity, including permanent pins-and-needles sensations in his hands and feet. Due to their toxicities, both of these medications had to be stopped. Paul was then off treatment for sixteen months, after which his bone marrow examination revealed progression of disease. Fortunately, in that interim off treatment, a new medication, just going through experimental trials at the time, was now available as an alternative. This new medication represented a major breakthrough in the treatment of this leukemia. It had few side effects compared to the older treatments, yet it was much more effective. It's now known as Gleevec.

Paul began on Gleevec in April 2001 and within six months the leukemia was again in remission. He has now been on Gleevec over twelve years and continues to do well. His last two bone marrow tests showed no evidence of the Philadelphia chromosome or other signs of leukemia. For now the leukemia specialists plan to keep him on it for good.

Paul continues to be very active though he has "semi-retired" from business and now works in state government. In retrospect it seems ironic to me that we were able to diagnose his leukemia the very moment it manifested itself - simply by taking the unusual path of monitoring blood counts for peptic ulcer disease as he did not want to "fool with stool" each month. What a blessing that turned out to be!

Malpractice

The "experts" tell us that the only physicians never sued for malpractice are those not involved in patient care. I suppose this means doctors who devote all their time to research or those employed by an insurance company. I am neither of those, so perhaps I should not have been surprised when I was sued for malpractice about twenty-five years ago. Though the patient herself did not want me to be named in the lawsuit by her lawyer, the lawyer filed suit against everyone involved in her care, including me. The circumstances of that case were quite unusual and make for an interesting story.

It was four in the morning when I received a call from the emergency room doctor. He reported that a patient of mine, Phyllis Johnson, had been brought in by ambulance semiconscious and moaning. He felt she had overdosed on her Ativan, a mild tranquilizer, and wanted to admit her to me. Oddly enough, at that time I had two patients named Phyllis Johnson. The younger was a woman in her late forties and the other a lady in her mid seventies, both of whom were taking low doses of Ativan for anxiety. I asked the ER doctor the age of the patient he was attending; he said he didn't know her age but that she was "old". He advised me he would admit her to the regular floor, and that it was reasonable for me to come to see her later in the morning. I told him I would see her at 7 a.m., and she was admitted. Unfortunately, he was wrong, both about which Phyllis Johnson he had admitted and about her diagnosis.

When I came to the hospital at 7 a.m. I saw right away that this was the younger Phyllis Johnson. This Phyllis I knew quite well. In her youth she had been involved with both alcohol and drug abuse. She was so proud that she had finally gotten away from that. Sadly, in order to get out from under the drug culture, she had to divorce her husband, who stubbornly refused to stop abusing drugs. When I met her, she was living on her own and working at a local factory. She very pleased to have her life back together. As she had some problems with mild anxiety that interfered with her daily life, I prescribed her a low dose of Ativan to help her with that. She was always very careful about its use, as she did not want to get back into a drug habit. When she was admitted, she had been using the Ativan very sparingly for almost a year. Thus I could not believe that she had overdosed on it.

On examining her I found she was unresponsive to voice or touch. With a mildly painful stimulus she would moan softly and move her arms or legs randomly. I immediately ordered a CAT scan of her brain to see if there was a more likely reason why she was so unresponsive. Unfortunately, the hospital's CAT scanner was not functioning. The radiologist assured me it would be repaired within an hour. An hour later, he again assured me it would be repaired in another hour. This went on through the morning and early afternoon, a delay of almost eight hours. Finally she had her CAT scan, which showed she had suffered an intracranial bleed from a leaking cerebral aneurysm. A cerebral aneurysm is a small sac-like projection off an artery. It can rupture much like a weak bulging spot on a car tire might blow out. In her case it had not completely blown but was leaking blood into her brain. It was this bleeding that had caused her loss of consciousness. I immediately arranged for her to be transported by helicopter to a neurosurgeon in the nearby large city. There she underwent surgery to remove the aneurysm. But for mild memory loss about the whole incident, she subsequently had a complete neurologic recovery.

Unfortunately, Phyllis still had a problem with the local hospital. Her insurance did not provide coverage for drug abuse or mental health problems, such as an overdose. They therefore denied payment for all of her local hospital care as her admitting diagnosis said, "Ativan overdose". When she had recovered, she arranged a meeting with the hospital administration and the ER doctor to try to resolve this issue so her insurance company would pay for her care. She asked if they would amend her record to show she was admitted for an intracranial bleed and not an overdose. However, the administration and the ER doctor refused to amend the record or even to send a letter to her insurance carrier explaining the situation. For this reason, she sought an attorney to bring a lawsuit against the hospital just for the cost of her care there.

As I mentioned previously, Phyllis' attorney decided to name everybody involved in her care in this lawsuit. Phyllis came to me to let me know she did not want me involved in the lawsuit as she felt I had saved her life, and we had always had a very good doctor-patient relationship. Her attorney nonetheless sued me as well. Unfortunately, the amount for which I was being sued was so small that my insurance company decided to settle the case for that amount; it was at least eight to ten times less than the cost of a legal defense for me. My malpractice insurance company's attorneys assured me that my case was easily defensible, and that I had indeed not done anything wrong. They agreed I had done my best to get her the care she needed, the only complicating factor being the delay in obtaining the CAT scan, yet this had been beyond my control. Indeed, the attorneys assured me that I would be exonerated should the case come to court.

However, there was a clause in my malpractice insurance contract stating that the insurance company could settle out-of-court if they felt this was less expensive, regardless of my wishes in the matter. Since in my case the cost of legal defense would be many times the cost of settlement, they decided to settle. Now I would have a permanent black mark on my record with the National Practitioner Data Bank, a federal agency that keeps track of malpractice suits against physicians. That lawsuit is still the only mark on my record. I was permitted to submit my comments regarding the circumstances of that malpractice settlement, but I could never have it deleted from the Data Bank.

The most interesting part of the whole incident came almost twenty years later, long after I had moved to another state to practice medicine. A surgical colleague and very close friend in that town had passed away. My wife, Diane, and I returned there for his funeral and to be with his widow for a few days. The four of us had all been good friends, and our children had grown up together. After the funeral we accompanied her to a restaurant to grieve and reminisce together, away from the large funeral crowd. While we were at the restaurant, a waitress came running toward us, her arms thrown wide, with a big smile on her face. It was Phyllis. She rushed up to give me a big hug, saying, "Oh, Dr. Yarbrough, I'm so glad to see you! You saved my life! You're the best doctor I've ever had!" She went on the tell everyone at our table how grateful she was that I had diagnosed her problem correctly and saved her life. I thanked her as graciously as I could, but I could not help feeling a bit uncomfortable as she was the only patient who had ever sued me in my entire professional career. It seemed ironic that she should be so warm and grateful for the care I had provided. Sometimes life just doesn't make sense.

Mama Knows Best

About three years ago I first saw Juanita, a pleasant twenty-two year-old girl who had recently moved from Mexico and was working as a waitress in one of the local Mexican restaurants. She initially came to me with complaint of unexplained weight loss, nocturnal sweats and fevers, loss of appetite (anorexia), and cough productive of small amounts of green mucus. Fortunately, she had never coughed up any blood. She said she developed these symptoms over the last few months while working at the restaurant. She insisted she had never had this problem in Mexico. She said that she had come here on a work visa to earn money to send back home to help out her family. Juanita told me she had been working sixty to eighty hours, seven days a week. She said that when she had first come here, she weighed 135 pounds, but now she was down to 117 pounds. Clearly, she was not doing well.

On examination I found she was congested with fluid behind her eardrums. Her nose showed red, swollen nasal turbinates consistent with sinusitis, and she had red sinus drainage tracks down the back of her throat, also indicating a sinus infection. Much to my surprise, the remainder of her examination was normal. Her chest was completely clear of congestion or other abnormality. It was obvious, though, that she was extremely fatigued. The presence of a sinus infection could explain her cough and fevers, but I felt there might be more to this.

After I finished examining her, I asked Juanita for more information about her background and how she was doing. Apparently, she was sleeping only four to six hours a night and eating very little. Indeed, she often skipped meals due to her work. Since Mexico has one of the world's highest prevalence rates for tuberculosis, my biggest concern was that Juanita might have it. The classic signs of tuberculosis include weight loss, anorexia, fever, cough, and night sweats, all of which she had. The bloody sputum associated with tuberculosis may not be present early in the disease. But before giving her a TB skin test, I had to find out if Juanita had been given BCG vaccine as a child.

The letters BCG stand for "Bacillus Calmette-Guérin". It is a vaccine against tuberculosis prepared from a strain of tubercular bacteria that infects cows. It is treated so it does not cause disease in humans but can produce immunity against the human tubercular bacillus. BCG vaccine is effective up to eighty percent of the time in preventing tuberculosis for as long as fifteen years. However, it seems to be less effective the closer one lives to the equator, and it's efficacy depends very much on which laboratory prepared the vaccine strain. BCG is particularly effective in preventing tuberculous meningitis in small children, but it's effectiveness against pulmonary tuberculosis is variable, especially in adults. For this reason a few countries, including the United States, have never used BCG routinely. It is felt that a reliable TB skin test to detect active disease is more useful. In addition, a previous

BCG vaccine can cause a severe, and falsely positive, TB skin test.

This is why it was so important to find out if Juanita had received BCG vaccine as an infant so we did not cause her to have a severe reaction with a TB skin test. When I asked if she knew whether or not she had received BCG vaccination as an infant in Mexico twenty-two years ago, Juanita told me she did not know. However, at our local hospital we had a hospitalist physician, a specialist in internal medicine, who was a very avid user of computers and the Internet. I called him and asked if he could find out whether indeed BCG had been given to infants in Mexico twenty-two years prior. He assured me he was certain he would be able to find the information I needed in just a few minutes of searching the Internet. He promised to call me back shortly.

As he had not called me back after a quarter hour, I decided to go ahead with treatment for Juanita's sinus infection, which I knew for certain that she did have. I prescribed an antibiotic, a mild decongestant, and a cough syrup with codeine, the last with the hope that she might at least get more sleep. I also advised her to try to cut back on her work hours so she could get more rest due to her fatigue. She seemed quite grateful for my helping her and prepared to leave.

Yet just before she walked out of the exam room, another thought occurred to me. I asked Juanita if she had ever talked with her mother since coming to the United States. She then told me that she spoke with her mother every evening. I asked if her mother would be home now, and she said that she probably was. I led Juanita to one of my office telephones and requested her to call her mother and ask whether she had received BCG vaccination as an infant. Her mother was indeed home, and she informed us that Juanita received BCG in the hospital right after her birth before she even went home with her mother. Now I knew we had done the right thing in not just giving her a TB skin test.

About two hours after Juanita had left, I received a call back from a very frustrated hospitalist. He told me he had tried to find the information on the Internet directly without success. He even searched the extensive Centers for Disease Control web site without finding an answer about Mexican practices so long ago. Finally, he told me that he had sent e-mails to all the infectious disease and internal medicine professors under whom he had trained to see if they could find this information and pass it along to us. He was shocked to find out that I had already learned the answer to my question. "How did you find out so fast?" he asked me. I replied, "It was simple. We used an 1885 technology, the telephone, and called her Mama in Mexico. She gave us the answer. They were giving BCG in Mexico twenty-two years ago." I could hear the hospitalist pound his fist on his desk as he said to me, "That's cheating!" As

I told him, "Well, sometimes the old technology beats the new."

Two weeks later Juanita was waiting on my wife and me in the restaurant where she worked. She told me she was gaining weight back, her appetite had returned, and she no longer had nocturnal fevers or sweats after taking the medication for her sinusitis. She also said she was very grateful to know never to have a TB skin test since she had received BCG as an infant. Old technology or new, sometimes Mama still knows best!

Motorcycle CPA

Growing up, John was always the last to be picked for sides in a sports game. Though he loved sports, he was soft and pudgy, with ruddy cheeks, wire-rim glasses, and a very studious personality. Nonetheless, he played sports whenever he could in grade school, high school, and college. Psychologists would call that a reaction formation, an increased interest and activity in an area where a person feels deficient, sometimes referred to as a "Napoleon complex". In John's case, though, he simply loved sports almost as much as he loved school.

John was still somewhat pudgy, with ruddy cheeks, and still wore the same wire-rim glasses when I first met him, but now he was bald but for a small ring of hair, closely cropped to his scalp. He certainly look the part of the CPA that he was, with an MBA, a wife, and two grown sons who loved sports just as much as their father. During the week John worked as an accountant, who, surprisingly, transformed into an avid motorcyclist on the weekends, riding his customized Harley-Davidson with the other members of his motorcycle club. It was, in a way, due to his motorcycle that John first came to see me. The weekend before John had noticed he was having weakness in his left ankle that gave him trouble shifting the gears on his Harley. John told me he had never had an ankle sprain or other injury in spite of playing sports most of his life, and he could not explain why he was now having trouble using his left ankle and foot to operate the gearshift lever on his bike.

After learning about John, as described above, I began to examine him. I found that the strength on flexion and extension of his left ankle was remarkably weak, yet there was no swelling, tenderness, or other sign of injury. Also, his left ankle and knee reflexes were both abnormally brisk, especially compared to his right ankle and knee. Though his sensation was intact, John had absolutely no pain. Were his problem due to a pinched nerve in his back from a bulging or herniated disc, I would have expected John to have a sciatica-type pain, yet he was pain-free. I also found that John's left calf muscles were softer, with less resting muscle tone, compared to the muscles of his right calf. Given these findings, I was suspicious that John had some type of neurologic injury or disease. I scheduled him for EMG/NCS (electromyography and nerve conduction study, respectively) and a subsequent visit with our local neurologist. Unfortunately, the neurologist confirmed what I had suspected. This was very probably Lou Gehrig's disease, amyotrophic lateral sclerosis, abbreviated ALS. Since John's symptoms only involved one body area, this diagnosis could not be certain, but it was suspected. Time would tell.

Amyotrophic lateral sclerosis is a degenerative disease of the nervous system which destroys the nerve cells in the motor cortex, the part of the brain which controls movement. It also involves spinal motor nerve cells as well as nerve cells in the bulbar - or hind brain - region. The body parts where the disease first appears and the rate of progression of the disease are both widely variable and probably determined by multiple different factors. ALS tends to predominate in men up to about age seventy; after that it seems to be equal in both sexes. Specialists feel that the actual onset of the disease very likely precedes the onset of the patient's symptoms by several years. The diagnosis is made through repeated clinical examinations rather than through multiple different tests. Today there is treatment available which seems to slow the progression of disease for some patients, but this was not available at the time John was diagnosed. Both MRI and PET scans can now contribute to the diagnosis, yet even today ALS is still primarily a clinical diagnosis, made by repeated examinations as the disease progresses and more deficits emerge. A definite diagnosis of ALS requires both upper motor neuron disease in the motor cortex and the bulbar area and lower motor neuron signs in the spinal area. There is still no cure; it is always fatal.

As weeks and then months went by, John found he was no longer able to ride his Harley. He now had a left flat-footed gait. We had him fitted with a brace behind his left heel and ankle, extending up the calf, to prevent foot drop. The brace enabled him to continue walking fairly well, but he was not able to shift the gears in his motorcycle any longer. Within six months of my having first met him, John then began having trouble with his left hand. Being a right-handed gentleman, he could still write, but being a CPA, he used his left hand to work the keys on his calculator. This was a devastating loss for him, as he now had to have an assistant run the totals for him in his work or try to use his right hand and work much slower. Now there were two separate body areas affected by the disease.

Within another six months of the involvement of his left hand, John began having slurring of his speech. At this time the neurologist confirmed a definite diagnosis of ALS. Unfortunately, the only treatment available to John was supportive. He now wore a brace on both his left foot and left hand. We referred him to a speech therapist to help him speak more clearly, but in spite of the therapy, his speech slowly worsened. Within fifteen months of his initial diagnosis, John had become dependent on a wheelchair most of the time for getting around his home. He had stopped working and was applying for disability.

I had a long talk with John and his wife; they agreed that he did not want to go on a ventilator or other life support system. We discussed a feeding tube since he was starting to have trouble swallowing. CPAP, or continuous positive airway pressure, similar to that used for sleep apnea, would help with his breathing as the disease began involving the diaphragm and intercostal muscles, the muscles of breathing. He declined both. John told me he understood his disease was relentlessly progressive and would ultimately result in his death. He told me he had discussed this with his wife and pastor; he was resigned to his fate.

He had made arrangements for his wife and children to be taken care of upon his death, and he did not want to prolong his life or their suffering. When he began having difficulty breathing, he indicated to me that he was now ready to go on hospice. We consulted hospice to provide him with terminal care. Within two years of his initial diagnosis, John had died.

My entire office staff had come to know John and to admire his courage in facing the disease with which he was afflicted. We therefore decided to close the office so that all of us could attend his funeral. There was a beautiful service at his church with his entire family present along with several hundred others. Apparently John's cycle club was part of a large consortium of motorcycle clubs. I had never seen so many motorcycles at one time. There must have been over two hundred of them leading the hearse to the cemetery where John was interred. Though only fifty-two years of age at his passing, John had lived a full life, enjoying all the sports that he loved, his vocation as a CPA, and his avocation as a motorcyclist. All of us would miss him.

Muscular Dystrophy

Perhaps the saddest case in my years of medical practice involved a little boy named Billy. I first saw Billy when he was six years old. His mother said he had complained of leg pain after playing on stairs at a relative's house. As far as she knew, he had not fallen or otherwise hurt himself, but she brought him to me just in case he had "done something to himself".

On careful examination I could not reproduce the pain in his leg that Billy's mother said he'd been complaining about. Billy would laugh and giggle as I touched the affected leg and even tell me he hurt when I touched him there. However, he told me the same thing if I merely touched his earlobe lightly. Given these findings, I advised his mother to give him ibuprofen only if he seemed to be in pain, at least until the pediatric orthopedist saw him.

At that office visit I noticed Billy also had a problem with his feet turning out more than 45°. His mother had taken him to a podiatrist who fitted him with shoe inserts, but this did not seem to help. When I first saw him he already had an appointment to see a pediatric orthopedist, a bone specialist, at the nearby university medical center. In addition to seeing how Billy's feet turned out, I also noted how he walked with a wide-based waddling gait, like a Charlie Chaplin walk. Also, his calf muscles were abnormally large and his thigh muscles seemed abnormally small in comparison. Finally, he was quite small overall for boys his age, though just inside the range of normal. All of these findings suggested Duchenne-type muscular dystrophy. I advised Billy's mother of my concerns, but I think she dismissed the idea as too awful to consider seriously.

The term dystrophy means abnormal growth. Duchenne-type muscular dystrophy, the most common hereditary neuromuscular disease, is characterized by enlargement of the calf muscles, progressive generalized muscular weakness, intellectual impairment, cardiac muscle involvement, and the proliferation of connective tissue and fat in the muscle. This disease is transmitted as an X-linked recessive trait, meaning it is inherited from the mother on the X chromosome. This occurs in about one out of 3,600 of male infants. It was in 1861 that Dr. Duquesne first characterized the features this illness, and his name subsequently became associated with it. There are several other types of muscular dystrophy, each with a different genetic transmission and clinical course. Some lead to death in infancy while others may be associated with a normal life span.

In Duchenne-type muscular dystrophy the boys rarely show symptoms until they are of toddler age. Early muscular skills such as rolling over, sitting, and standing, are usually achieved at an appropriate age. These boys usually begin walking at the normal age of one year, though walking may be slightly delayed; Billy did not walk until he was fifteen months old. Subtle muscle weakness may be seen in some affected boys as early as two years of age. Because the onset of muscle weakness predominately affects hip and upper leg muscles, these boys use the arms and hands to help them "climb up" on one leg to get up from sitting on the floor. This is known as Gower's sign, and it can almost always be seen by the time the affected boy is five or six years old. This sign was already present when I first saw Billy. The characteristic waddling gait also usually appears about this age, and Billy had it.

The pediatric orthopedist performed a muscle biopsy on Billy, which has been the gold standard for diagnosis of muscular dystrophy since the 1860s. Unfortunately, the biopsy confirmed the diagnosis. The orthopedist referred Billy to the Muscular Dystrophy Clinic. At their first visit to that clinic the family was informed of what to expect from this illness. The clinic examination noted Billy's waddling gait, the Gower's sign, and marked weakness in the hip, pelvis, and shoulder muscles. His family was informed that there was no specific treatment available to halt or reverse the disease, and that by the time most of these boys are teens, they can no longer walk and are wheelchair bound. After answering his parents' questions in as much detail as possible, the neurologist scheduled Billy to be seen by a pediatric cardiologist for a baseline evaluation and then for his return visit to their clinic.

Sadly, before Billy reached age ten, he was no longer able to walk. The loss of the ability to walk is devastating not only psychologically but physically as well. Being able to walk will postpone the gradual onset of osteoporosis, thinning of the bones from disuse. This can get so severe that these boys just bump into stationary objects with their wheelchairs and sustain fractures due to the fragility of their thin bones.

With loss of the ability to walk they also develop thoracolumbar scoliosis, a side-to-side S-shaped curvature of the spine, which becomes rapidly progressive in muscular dystrophy once the boy is wheelchair bound. As the degree of scoliotic curvature worsens, this can compress one of the lungs as well as the heart. The scoliosis may then require major back surgery to correct the dangerous curvature.

In addition, due to the lack of normal movement, there are often contractures involving the ankles, knees, hips, and elbows. These contractures dramatically limit the mobility of those joints and thus the patient's ability to continue functioning as normally as possible. As the disease progresses, it can involve the muscles of breathing, resulting in a weak and ineffective cough and frequent pneumonia. Fortunately, the child is usually able to continue to use a pencil, eating utensils, and a computer keyboard.

While there is intellectual impairment in all muscular dystrophy patients, usually it is fairly minor. Most of these boys have relatively mild learning disabilities and are still able to function in a regular classroom. What seems surprising is how cheerful the affected children seem to be even though they must deal with such severe disability and early death. Billy would always smile at me with a shy grin whenever we would see each other.

Although this disorder also involves the muscle of the heart, the cardiac involvement does not always correspond to the skeletal muscle involvement. Some patients die from severe cardiac muscle disease while still able to walk. Others, who are in the final stages of the muscular disease, still have good heart function. The average life span for these boys is eighteen years. Most often they die from end-stage heart failure or respiratory failure in their sleep. Occasionally, a severe pneumonia leads to their death.

Since the specialists now provided most of his care, I would see Billy more often in church than in the office. For the first few years he would try to walk, but it didn't seem long before he attended church in his power wheelchair. The last few years I have not seen him. About five years ago his parents changed insurance, and I was not a "preferred provider" on that new insurance. He must now be in his late teens and nearing the end of his expected life span.

Billy's was truly one of the saddest cases I have ever been involved with as a family physician. In trying to help Billy and his family deal with this disorder, I could understand how the family doctor of a hundred years ago must have felt. The doctor back then could diagnose very well but had little treatment to offer. Most of the time all the doctor could do was let the family know what to expect from a given illness, and how long it would take to run its course. As Billy's physician, I found this to be a very helpless feeling. I wanted to do more for Billy, but there was nothing more that could be done in confronting this terrible disease.

Normal Pressure Hydrocephalus

Henry had had interesting life. He grew up on a farm just a few miles from town with no electricity or indoor plumbing. However, days after the bombing of Pearl Harbor on December 7, 1941, he said "goodbye" to his family and girlfriend; Henry had enlisted in the Navy. He was trained as a radioman in the service, and during World War II he served on a variety of different naval vessels as their radio operator. Once he told me two of those ships had been sunk from underneath him during the war. After the war he left the Navy and returned home. Back home the only job he could find that would utilize his training was as a telegrapher for the railroad, a position he held until retirement. He told me that in his later years with the railroad, they used radios instead of the telegraph, but he didn't mind. He had already developed a strong ham radio and short-wave habit, listening and talking with like-minded people all over the world. He also was an avid hunter and fisherman in his spare time. Henry liked to stay busy.

When I first met Henry, he was a tall, lean, angular gentleman of seventy-two years with a full shock of light sandy-brown hair and pale blue eyes. I saw him initially for high cholesterol and neuropathy with burning, tingling sensations in his feet and lower legs. Henry thought this was likely due to the medication he had been taking for his cholesterol, but simple blood tests proved it was from B-12 deficiency. He was begun on B-12 shots weekly at first, then monthly, and his symptoms resolved. After that I saw him regularly every three months to check on his cholesterol and blood pressure, along with an annual prostate check. Henry was a joy to take care of as he always watched his weight and diet, exercised regularly, and kept his cholesterol under excellent control.

Unfortunately, about four years after I first met him, Henry began having trouble with memory and then with walking. He became progressively more unsteady on his feet and had several falls. He began walking with a cane. Within six months he progressively worsened to where he was walking with tiny steps in a shuffling gait, very dependent upon the walker he had finally begun using. Now he had lost the ability to drive. I checked an MRI of his lower back, but it showed no abnormalities to explain this. In addition, he started having worsening memory problems. At first, it was just trying to remember the call letters of some of his frequent ham radio contacts. Yet within a few months, Henry would shuffle into the kitchen and forget why he had gone there. Finally, it got to the point that he could not remember how to get home from the grocery store.

As his walking and memory worsened, Henry also starting having a tremor such that by the time he had to start using a walker, he could not sip a cup of coffee without spilling it on himself. I referred him to our local neurologist, who thought he might have Parkinson's disease causing the tremor and the trouble walking. He prescribed medicine for Parkinson disease, but it was of no help. Finally, Henry developed difficulty controlling his urine. At this point, his wife was considering nursing home placement for Henry, something he had never wanted to do.

When Henry's wife told me about the urinary troubles, I became very suspicious that Henry might have normal pressure hydrocephalus, or NPH. I ordered a CAT scan of his head, and unlike the MRI of his lumbar spine, this was markedly abnormal. The CAT scan showed that Henry's ventricles, the chambers in the brain filled with cerebrospinal fluid, were dramatically enlarged. Henry's gait disturbance, dementia, urinary trouble, and now enlarged ventricles, confirmed my suspicion that he had NPH.

Normal pressure hydrocephalus is a disorder that usually shows up after age sixty, but occasionally it can start at a younger age. Hydrocephalus, often known as "water on the brain", refers to a large amount of

cerebrospinal fluid present within the head. In this disease the excess is in the ventricles within the brain. In addition, the term "normal pressure" is misleading. Although the fluid pressure seems normal, it does exert pressure on the soft brain tissues so that over time the ventricles become greatly enlarged. The cause of normal pressure hydrocephalus is not known. The disorder produces the triad of symptoms of gait problems, a dementia resembling

Alzheimer's, and difficulty in controlling urination. Some patients, such as Henry, will even develop a tremor suggesting Parkinson's disease.

To test Henry for NPH, I performed a spinal tap on him and removed 30 cc, or one ounce, of spinal fluid. His gait disturbance improved temporarily, suggesting that Henry was suffering from NPH. Yet when I discussed his case with the neurosurgeon, he wasn't so sure. The neurosurgeon agreed to see Henry in consultation and then scheduled him for a four-day cisternogram test. In this test a radioactive tracer is injected into the spinal fluid. In normal patients the tracer will be distributed in most of the spinal fluid but not in the ventricles; it remains detectable only one or two days. In patients with NPH, the radioactive tracer will reflux up into the ventricles and persist there for two or more days, which it did in Henry's test. The neurosurgeon then agreed with me that Henry had NPH and would likely benefit from having a shunt. He scheduled Henry for a shunt placement the next day.

A shunt is a small plastic tubing with a one-way pressure valve that is placed into one of the ventricles, then passed down under the skin into the peritoneal space within the abdomen, where the excess fluid can be harmlessly absorbed. The pressure gradient across the one-way valve can usually be adjusted without repeat surgery, as needed according to the patient's response and clinical status.

Within two weeks of the shunt placement Henry's trouble with walking and urination had completely disappeared. A month after receiving the shunt, Henry's Alzheimer's-like dementia was completely gone, his memory having fully returned. He was now able to drive, operate his ham radio, and even resume fishing trips. Unfortunately, the only symptom that did not fully resolve was the tremor in his hands, which made it difficult to drink a cup of coffee, eat peas with a fork, or sign his name. Fortunately, with the addition of a beta-blocker medication, the tremor diminished to the point that he could perform these tasks easily again.

The complete resolution of dementia, trouble walking, and urinary symptoms was extremely dramatic for Henry. Sadly, it is estimated that a small percentage of the patients in nursing homes around the country are afflicted with NPH, as Henry had been, but are misdiagnosed as having Parkinson's or Alzheimer's disease. I can't help but wonder how many could be restored to their normal lives if those patients with enlarged ventricles, stumbling gait, urinary incontinence, and dementia were all investigated for NPH. To me, saving even a few of them from so awful a fate would be worth the cost of screening them for this. Henry would agree.

Paracentesis

"Can you help my father?" These were the first words from Lois, an elementary school administrator in her early thirties. Lois was a very trim, professional looking lady with shoulder length reddish-brown hair wearing a deep blue dress with a white sash and collar. She taken the morning off from her job for an appointment she had scheduled with me to talk about her father. She seemed quite professional and composed sitting across from me, but one could see tears welling up in her eyes as she began telling me of her father, George, only fifty-nine years old, who was dying with pancreatic cancer.

George had been a hard-working rancher, whose ranch was just outside of town. There he raised Angus cattle and six daughters, the youngest of which was telling me his story. About nine months before, he had begun feeling fatigued. Like most farmers and ranchers, he finally went to the doctor but only under protest. The doctor tested him for anemia, thyroid disease, B12 deficiency, and ordered a general chemistry panel looking for common causes of fatigue. All the tests were normal. The doctor then advised George to get more rest and see if this would not resolve his fatigue. It did not.

Three months later he began having vague abdominal pain between his rib margin and bellybutton, the epigastric area. Again, reluctantly, he went to the doctor and was diagnosed with gastritis and given a prescription for Prilosec, a medication to reduce stomach acid production and release. No tests were done at this time. The doctor advised George that this medicine should help, but if his symptoms continued, he was to return for further evaluation and testing. George took the medication for about two weeks. It seemed to help a little at first, but then it seemed to stop working, so George stopped taking it.

Next his wife of forty years noticed that George was not eating much. He passed it off as just not having much appetite. As a result, over the next few months he began losing what would become a dramatic amount of weight. Concerned about her husband, she called their youngest daughter, looking for help to convince George to return to the doctor. He finally agreed, and the doctor decided more investigation was needed. He scheduled George for a CT scan of the abdomen, which, unfortunately, showed a large mass in the pancreas, dozens of tumor growths in the liver, and hundreds of tiny implants of tumor throughout the abdomen. George was then scheduled for a CT-directed needle biopsy of one of the lesions in his liver. This showed that George had widespread metastatic cancer of the pancreas. His doctor then referred George to an oncologist who told him that little could be done at this advanced stage of the disease. He advised George to contact a local hospice for comfort care.

Lois, his daughter, told me that her father had been on hospice about six weeks. She felt his current doctor had lost interest in helping him. When asked what she meant by that, she told me George had developed large quantities of fluid in his abdomen which made it difficult for him to breathe. He had received a paracentesis during a short respite hospital stay about three weeks ago, and that gave him dramatic help in breathing much better. However, the fluid had now re-accumulated such that George was breathing in rapid shallow gasps. His current doctor was unwilling to repeat the paracentesis as an outpatient in his office, and she was asking if I would consider doing it in my office to relieve her father's discomfort and shortness of breath.

Pancreatic cancer is the fourth most common cause of cancer deaths in this country though its incidence is rather low. This is because, as was the case with George, this type of cancer is not usually detected until late in the disease process. Symptoms from this are often very vague or even absent early in the disease. The five-year survival rate for pancreatic cancer is less than five percent. Most patients die within the first two years after diagnosis. At times the first sign of these cancers is seen in the patient's eyes as they begin turning yellow with jaundice from obstruction of the common bile duct by the growth of the cancer around it. By this time the cancer is usually widespread with implants throughout the abdomen and in the liver. As in George's case, these tumors produce free fluid in the abdomen, known as ascites, causing swelling of the abdomen, often with significant pain and difficulty breathing from the pressure.

In some cases reducing salt and fluid intake and may help to relieve the pressure of ascites. For some patients diuretics can be used to get the kidneys to excrete some of the excess fluid, but their use is limited by the low blood pressure these patients often have. Thus, as was the case with George, paracentesis may offer the only real relief from this problem. Although ascites can be monitored by serial measurements of the abdominal girth or weight, the most useful indicator for the need for paracentesis in patients like George is the patient's progressive shortness or breath.

Paracentesis gives good, though temporary, symptom relief. To do this procedure the doctor will percuss, or tap on his fingers as they touch the abdomen, to find the level where the sound changes from hollow and reverberating to dull and non-echoing. That change in sound marks the level of the ascites fluid in the abdomen. Below this line the skin is prepped with an antiseptic and injected with a local anesthetic. A large intravenous-type catheter is next inserted into the abdomen, the needle then withdrawn leaving the catheter in place. This is connected to IV tubing attached to collection bottles, and three or four liters of fluid are thus removed. This results in dramatic relief of the pressure discomfort and shortness of breath the patient was experiencing. There are risks to the procedure including the development of spontaneous bacterial peritonitis, bleeding, and, if percussion is not done correctly, perforation of a bowel loop. Often the patient is given antibiotics prophylactically to prevent spontaneous bacterial peritonitis.

I assured Lois I would begin that very day doing periodic paracentesis in the office to relieve her father's discomfort. The first time he came in, it was obvious that George had been a big muscular man, the typical mental picture one might have of a hard-working rancher. However, he now looked nine months pregnant, perhaps with twins. He clearly had lost a substantial amount of his body weight and was extremely short of breath. Prior to the paracentesis we had had George take an oral antibiotic to reduce his risk of infection. We could then proceed right away with the paracentesis procedure, the first time removing four liters of fluid. Upon completion of this, George was dramatically better, breathing comfortably for the first time in weeks. George asked me when he could have this done again, and I advised him the timing for this procedure was dependent entirely upon him and his breathing. When he felt too short of breath to put up with it any longer, he was to have someone call to schedule another paracentesis, which I promised we would do either that day or the next.

For four months we did periodic paracenteses for George, each time removing between three and four liters of fluid, each time giving him rather dramatic relief from his shortness of breath. He understood that this would not prolong his life, but it would provide him greater comfort a during the dying process. He accepted this and was grateful that we were able to give him another four months with his family. Lois told me that during that time his temperament softened, and in his final days George was able to let everyone in the immediate family know that he loved them and tried to comfort them in their grief. He passed away in his sleep at home.

Lois has always been grateful that we provided her father with this service during his last months. Now, long after George's passing, there is a new procedure called transjugular intrahepatic portosystemic shunt, or TIPS for short. This can be done for patients with severe recurrent ascites such as George had. This new procedure appears to be more effective at removing excess ascites as compared to paracentesis, and there is no significant difference in complications, such as bleeding or infection. TIPS may offer even greater relief in the future for patients with ascites like George.

Perfect Care

Peter and Haley were the "perfect" couple. Both grew up in upper middle class families and were attractive, athletic young people. They attended the "best" schools, he becoming an MBA and she an attorney. With the completion of their education they had moved back to town. Peter became a bank vice-president and Haley the newest partner in the town's "best" and most well-established law firm. After working for five years to secure themselves financially in the manner to which they had been accustomed, they decide it was the perfect time to have a baby. Haley ceased taking her birth control pills, and within less than a year they had achieved a pregnancy.

Haley and Peter decided to seek obstetrical care from the "best" obstetrician, a member of a large, well-known medical clinic in town, and Haley selected that doctor's recommendation for the "best" pediatrician to care for the baby in the hospital. Haley was very careful with diet and exercise during her pregnancy. She was afraid to gain even the least bit of extra weight and was dismayed at the changes in her body with pregnancy. She and Peter were busy throughout her pregnancy making rather detailed plans for their baby's future. In her law practice Haley's partners made allowances for her as her pregnancy progressed, so that she was still able to carry a light workload in spite of being near term. Haley attended prepared childbirth classes, convinced she would sail through natural childbirth. On the Saturday before her due date, she was admitted to the hospital expecting to pass this "test" without problem. Unfortunately, childbirth is not as predictable as a college exam.

Although Haley followed all the prepared childbirth recommendations, with Peter at her side during her labor, she simply was unable to progress to vaginal delivery. Her trim figure may have been attractive in a dress, but her small pelvic size was not the best for childbirth. After a few hours of failure to progress, her obstetrician recommended a cesarean section. Her labor was on the Saturday of a holiday weekend, so a surgical crew had to be called in from home. In that hospital, cesarean sections were done in the OR, not on the OB unit. Also, a doctor had to be found to attend the newborn at the cesarean section. The baby doctor Haley had chosen was at the lake with her family and would not likely make it there in time. Several other physicians were called, but no one else was available, except for the ER physician - me.

At that hospital at that time, the ER physician was not allowed to leave the Emergency Department while on duty, even for meals. These had to be brought either from the hospital cafeteria or from home so the physician would be in constant attendance in the department. This, of course, conflicted with the needs of the obstetrician to have a doctor standing by for the baby at the impending cesarean section. Since no one else was available for the baby, I agreed to standby, as a last resort, for the initial care of the infant.

Once the surgical team arrived, the C-section proceeded without delay. The baby was delivered and handed to me, and I could see at once that the baby's initial respiratory efforts were slightly depressed. The baby's color was good, but his heartbeat was slightly slow. After suctioning the baby's mouth then nose, he still was not breathing vigorously. In addition he had what is called acrocyanosis, or blue color to his hands and feet. To assist the baby, I then provided bag ventilation. After thirty seconds of this the baby's color improved, and his breathing normalized. He now had a vigorous cry, and we transported him from the OR to the newborn nursery. The "best" pediatrician by then had arrived and assumed the baby's care. I returned immediately to the ER.

While Haley's recovery was uneventful, her baby's was not. His pediatrician noticed his breath sounds over the right lung were slightly less than on the left. She ordered a portable chest x-ray. This showed a small pneumothorax, or air around the right lung, but the baby appeared to be breathing well with normal color and heartbeat. Nonetheless, the pediatrician decided to insert a small IV catheter through the skin to aspirate out the pneumothorax. Unfortunately, when she did so, an air leak developed at the puncture site. This required the placement of a chest tube, which prolonged the baby's hospitalization an extra week.

As Haley was an attorney, she discussed what had happened with one of her colleagues. They decided to file a lawsuit against the hospital, the pediatrician, and myself for the "injury" to her infant, as this was not the perfect outcome Haley had expected. My involvement began with a subpoena for interrogatories, or questions, in front of the attorneys for Haley, the hospital, and me. I went to the meeting with my wife, an experienced OB nurse, and answered all their questions as best I could.

The first few questions were about my training. I had completed elective rotations in anesthesia as well as newborn nursery while a resident. I explained the proper method of ventilating a newborn baby, fifty to sixty times a minute with a self-inflating bag, at thirty to forty centimeters' water pressure, just enough to produce a slight rise in the baby's chest. With this proper ventilation, a baby's heart rate, color, muscle tone, and respiratory effort should all improve. Certainly there were no signs of respiratory distress when Haley and Peter's baby was admitted to the newborn nursery.

Moreover, it is not uncommon for small air leaks to develop spontaneously as the lungs of the newborn fill with air for the first time. The risk is, of course, greater if positive pressure ventilation is required. Yet such a small pneumothorax as this baby had would not cause problems with heartbeat or breathing and should resolve on its own. However, in this case, for some reason the pediatrician had decided to try to resolve it herself. I pointed out that the baby had required minimal ventilation assistance immediately after birth, and that with it the baby's heart rate and breathing had improved. Finally, the attorneys had no more questions.

At that point, my wife Dianne, an RN of many years' experience, then spoke up and said she had a question for the lawyers, who seemed annoyed at her request. Dianne then mentioned how she had to bring me meals when I worked the ER, as leaving the department was against the hospital's rules and regulations. Yet in this circumstance, there was no one else available to provide newborn care in the operating room. She then asked these lawyers if my actions would not therefore come under the Good Samaritan law, since I was doing what a reasonable physician would do in such an emergent situation, and I had never billed for the care I had provided. The hospital's and Haley's attorney looked wide-eyed at each other, then turned to Dianne and said in unison, "You're right." My attorney just smiled.

I was immediately dropped from the impending lawsuit, thanks to Dianne's timely remarks. Sadly, the hospital as well as the pediatrician both eventually had verdicts against them due to the pediatrician's decision to intervene for what appeared to have been a harmless pneumothorax, attempting perhaps to provide Haley and Peter with the perfect outcome they had expected. Medicine is both an art and a science, an endeavor over which no physician ever exerts full control. As Plato put it centuries ago, "The enemy of the Good is the Perfect."

Prior Authorization

For the last several years, I have been treating Lin, a short attractive Chinese lady, who looks much younger than her fifty years, for severe seasonal allergies. She is married to a retired Air Force officer, and so she had the insurance for retired military. The first year she came to me, she reported having had the classic itchy, watery eyes, runny nose, excessive sneezing, and postnasal drainage with cough so characteristic of allergic rhinitis. She said this happened only through the summer months. On examination I found her nasal turbinates, the folds covering the openings of the sinuses on the inner sides of the nose, were swollen and pale with a clear watery drainage. Her conjunctiva, the membranes covering the inside of the eyelids and extending onto the sclera (the white of the eye), were inflamed and quite red. She clearly had bad allergic rhinitis. I advised her to try three different antihistamines, Claritin (loratadine), Allegra (fexofenadine), or Zyrtec (cetirizine). She needed to find out which of these worked best for her, then use it that summer for her allergies. She thanked me very kindly and did not return until the following year.

That second year she said she had found last year that Allegra worked best for her. However, it still did not control her allergy symptoms completely. She asked if there was anything else she could try. I then advised Lin of the step-therapy approach to the treatment of allergies, beginning with an antihistamine as she had done, then next adding a corticosteroid nasal spray. I explained to her how an antihistamine blocks the effects of histamine released from mast cells, specialized cells in the body where histamine granules are stored. Now we would add Flonase, a corticosteroid nasal spray, which would stabilize the mast cells in the nasal mucous membranes to block the release of histamine in the first place. She agreed to try the nasal spray along with her Allegra, and once more she thanked me very politely. I saw her again later that year for a sinus infection, and at that time she told me the combination of Allegra and Flonase nasal spray helped her control her allergy symptoms much better than the preceding year.

Unfortunately, the following year we had very heavy spring rains followed by a drought which caused tremendous growth and pollen release by the plants in our area. Lin's allergies were now worse than ever. Lin again returned, this time wondering if there was anything else that could be done for her allergies. I advised her that the next step would be the addition of Singulair, a leukotriene receptor antagonist. These chemicals, leukotrienes, are released in the inflammatory process of both asthma and allergic rhinitis. Singulair is indicated for those over one year of age with asthma and over two years of age with seasonal allergic rhinitis. It can even be used down to six months of age for perennial allergic rhinitis, an allergy that lasts year round.

I explained to Lin how Singulair works by a third and different mechanism of action from the nasal spray and the antihistamine. With these three different medications, with three different mechanisms of action, her allergy symptoms should be much better. As it was fairly late in her allergy season when Lynn came into see me, I gave her enough samples of Singulair to last through the remainder of that year's allergy season. I asked her to call me in a week or two weeks to let me know how this new medication worked for her. She called in a week to say that she had absolutely no allergy symptoms now and could even do without the corticosteroid nasal spray.

The next year Lin came in late spring to get prescriptions for her allergies. As her antihistamine was over-the-counter now, I gave her new prescriptions for both Flonase nasal spray and the Singulair tablets. I wasn't sure if she might not need the nasal spray this year, though she hadn't toward the end of last year's allergy season. I wanted her to have that available to her in her medication arsenal. I felt that might be the last I heard from Lin through the summer, but that was not to be the case. I received a phone call from her pharmacist who said that her insurance required a prior authorization to cover Singulair. He printed out their form and had Lynn bring it to me. I immediately filled it out, explaining how she had tried step therapy and now needed Singulair. I sent in the form expecting prompt approval for her.

Unfortunately, her insurance sent both Lin and I a letter saying that they would not cover Singulair for the indication of allergies, but only for asthma. They did this in spite of the fact that this medication has an FDA indication for both conditions. The letter said we could appeal that decision, and Lin asked me to do so. I reviewed Lynn's chart that day and composed what I thought would be a very effective letter. I described how Lin had gone through the appropriate steps of therapy to bring her allergies under control. I specifically pointed out how she had done magnificently with the Singulair the preceding year, even being able to stop the use of a corticosteroid. I again sent this letter to her insurer expecting that they would review it and approve her medication.

The next Lin and I heard from her insurance was a letter stating that they still would not approve Singulair for coverage for the diagnosis of allergies. It seemed it had not mattered to them that the medication worked extremely well for her, nor did it matter to them that she was able to come off the corticosteroid by taking Singulair. They simply would not cover the medication for allergic rhinitis.

A month after we had both received the denial letter for coverage for Singulair, her insurer sent us each another letter. In that letter they suggested she return to me to get started with a corticosteroid metered dose inhaler for management of her asthma, since they could see that she had not been prescribed that type of medication before.

Both of us laughed at this letter, since we both knew that she had never had any wheezing or other signs of asthma.

The last episode of this story was the strangest of all. Lin finally decided to see a nearby allergist for desensitization shots for her allergies. It required her to be tested for various allergens to see which of them caused her an allergic reaction. Next a special serum had to be prepared, of which she had to receive weekly doses with gradually increasing concentration until she no longer had a reaction to those allergens. That process could result in severe reaction at any time with any one of the injections she would receive. She would have to wait in the doctor's office for at least twenty minutes after each injection to make sure she did not have a reaction. The desensitization process would cost over $2,000, take over a year to complete, and has only about a fifty percent success rate. This was clearly more hazardous and much more expensive than Singulair, but remarkably, as Lin later told me, her insurance would cover it.

Sometimes insurance company rules make no sense.

PSA

The PSA test measures prostate specific antigen, a protein not found in other body tissues. Its normal range is up to 4.00. The test has been much maligned recently, and some are even recommending it no longer be used. Yet when used properly, it is still a good test. It can be elevated in the presence of prostate enlargement, infection, injury, or cancer. Yet it can still be normal even when cancer is present. While the PSA by itself is often of little value, when combined with the digital rectal exam to check the size and consistency of the prostate, it can be very helpful, particularly as it changes over time. Three vignettes, all true, will show the value of a properly interpreted PSA.

Roger came to me as a patient the first year I came to Kansas. He had hypertension but wanted to see me for a prostate check. As he said, "Doc, my father and brother have both had prostate trouble, so I suppose I should get mine checked." Roger was in his mid fifties and had no problems to suggest prostate disease. He came in simply because of the problems of the other men in his family.

The first thing I did was have Roger get his PSA drawn. Examination of the prostate can falsely elevate this test, so it was important to have the blood drawn first. Once we had drawn the PSA, I performed the digital prostate exam. I found Roger's prostate to be minimally enlarged, but there was a suspicious hard spot at the apex of the gland. I informed him of this and advised him to have this spot biopsied by a urologist. He agreed. I arranged for him to see the urologist and rescheduled him later about his blood pressure. A few weeks later, I received a call from the urologist. Roger's biopsy showed a localized but highly aggressive cancer. Although Roger's PSA was only 2.32, the biopsy showed a very high Gleason score. The cancer was present in most of the ten tissue cores normally collected for prostate biopsy.

The Gleason score consists of two numbers, each scored from one to five, five being the most abnormal.

The first number represents the most common pattern seen on the biopsy, and the second number scores the most abnormal area seen. The two together are the Gleason score. In Roger's case, his score was 5+5 or 10, the worst score one could get, representing a highly abnormal and aggressive cancer.

When Roger discussed this finding with his wife, Jean, they decided to go to M.D. Anderson Hospital in Houston, Texas, a major cancer center. There Roger underwent a radical prostatectomy, the removal of the entire prostate gland. Fortunately, examination of the tissue removed at surgery documented that he had a complete surgical cure from this highly aggressive cancer. For the first month after surgery, Roger had to wear adult diapers, as he had lost control of his bladder. After that first month, though, bladder control came back. Because Roger came for screening early, we were able to diagnose his cancer and get him to appropriate treatment in time. It has now been over ten years since Roger's surgery, and he has had no cancer recurrence.

Gene had a very different story. He had no family history of prostate cancer, so he was not particularly concerned about having a prostate check. I urged him to have it done since he was 55 years old. He begrudgingly agreed. Once again, I found an abnormal hard spot on prostate exam. Unlike Roger, Gene's PSA was 8.55, clearly elevated, though the gland was hardly enlarged. Gene's biopsy revealed the presence of prostate cancer, but in his case the Gleason score was only 1 + 2, or 3 total. Also, the cancer was present in only one of the ten standard biopsy specimens.

With these findings there was no urgency to proceed with any surgery, as Roger had had done. Rather, for the last five years, Gene has made regular visits to the urologist, who continues to monitor his PSA, clinical prostate exam, and sometimes an ultrasound of the prostate. This monitoring has proven that Gene's cancer has not progressed and, indeed, been very stable. This prostate cancer is very unlikely to cause death. In Gene's case, careful monitoring and watchful waiting are appropriate. Gene does not want to have surgery unless absolutely necessary, and he is pleased that his cancer is so slow-growing.

Over the past several years Gene's PSA has varied between 7.00 to 9.00. Most of the results have been about twice the upper limit of normal. Yet when this abnormal PSA is considered in light of the Gleason score from the biopsy, coupled with findings of repeated examinations, there is clearly no reason to recommend any more aggressive treatment for Gene.

Frank's story was altogether different. Frank had retired in Texas after working over thirty years as a baker. He and his wife Dorothy had planned to make their retirement in Texas, but their adult children were "driving them crazy". To get away from the children, they decided to move here, where Dorothy had grown up. She insisted, however, that Frank see a doctor to get "some arthritis pills". He had been having progressively increasing pain for almost a year, which she was sure was from arthritis.

When Frank came to see me shortly after moving into their new home, he brought with him his medical records from Texas. He explained that being just two months shy of going on Medicare, he didn't want something too expensive. I quickly reviewed Frank's records and found that his PSA had been rising progressively over several years. The most recent, done just six months prior was 13.5, and when I asked Frank where his pain hurt the worst that day, he pointed to the middle of his upper arm!

On digital rectal examination, I discovered Frank's prostate was greatly enlarged, the size of an average lemon, and the entire gland was rock hard. Clearly this was prostate cancer, and just as clearly, Frank's pain was not arthritis, but pain from the spread of prostate cancer to his bones. When I explained all this to Frank, he began to get tears in his eyes and, shaking in anger and shock, asked, "Why didn't that doctor in Texas ever check me like you just did?" I told him I could not answer that question.

I advised Frank that I would give him a big shot of long-acting cortisone to suppress the severe bone inflammation and hopefully lessen his pain. I also prescribed some strong pain pills should he need them. Neither of these two measures were expensive, and together they should tide him over until he went on Medicare and could afford to see the urologist. Two months later I received the results of the bone scan that the urologist had ordered for Frank. It showed evidence of prostate cancer in nearly every one of his bones. Frank died six weeks later.

These three stories illustrate that it is a combination of factors - among them the PSA, findings on digital rectal exam, and the Gleason score on prostate biopsies - that can lead to an informed decision about what to do in each individual case. Though many experts are recommending that the PSA be abandoned, I still feel it can be a helpful test. For Roger, the PSA could have given false reassurance that all was well. For Gene, serial PSA tests have assured his urologist and him that watchful monitoring is appropriate. For Frank, the rising PSA was an unheeded warning that more should have been done. To abandon the PSA test seems to me to be like throwing away a golf club because the one who owns can't hit a good golf ball. The problem is not in the instrument but rather in how it's used. Hopefully, the PSA will continue to be available as just one of many tools for evaluating prostate disease.

Pulmonary Hypertension

Born in the depths of the depression, Maddy was raised on a farm outside of town where they at least had enough to eat through those lean years. Maddy had always been somewhat of a rebel, starting dating and smoking cigarettes at age sixteen, much to her parents dismay. By age eighteen Maddy was a lean, buxom blonde girl, quite attractive, who decided to go her own way, and left for the big city with her best girlfriend from high school, who was also somewhat of a rebel. Neither of them could wait to get away from the farm to the bright lights and activities of the big-city. Maddy took a job at a factory and worked there for the first few years, sharing an apartment with her best friend.

Soon Maddy met Ralph, who ran his own heating business, and often came to the factory where Maddy worked to repair the furnaces and radiators. It was on one of those service calls that Ralph first met Maddy while she was on a break. He asked her out, and eventually they fell in love, married, and raised three children in the city. After many years in the city, Ralph was ready to retire. Though they had always expected to stay in the big city, there was a problem with that plan. Maddy had continued to smoke. By the time Ralph retired, she could no longer stand the city air pollution. They decided to return to the small-town where Maddy had attended high school, as her chronic obstructive pulmonary disease, COPD, had become so severe.

Chronic obstructive pulmonary disease is the preferred term for both chronic bronchitis and emphysema since most patients with COPD have both airspace destruction (emphysema), and airway changes (chronic bronchitis). Smoking is the main risk factor for COPD, now the fourth leading cause of death in the United States. The number of women affected now exceeds the number of men. In addition to tobacco use, years of exposure to very dusty work environments, such as mines, cotton mills, and grain facilities, may contribute to COPD. Air pollution was once thought to be a cause, but we now know that pre-existing of COPD, such as Maddy had, is what contributes to the ill effects of smog.

The emphysema part of COPD is characterized by destruction of the walls separating lung air sacs, or alveoli, leading to the development of large air sacs called blebs. Geometry tells us that the smaller a ball is, the greater its surface area relative to its diameter. As a result, when the tiny alveoli coalesce to form large blebs, there is much less surface area available for the exchange of oxygen and carbon dioxide, leading to shortness of breath, lower blood oxygen and higher blood carbon dioxide. The chronic bronchitis part of COPD is characterized by the enlargement of the bronchial mucous glands, destruction of the tiny cilia, the hair-like fibers on the bronchial lining cells that help sweep out mucus, and spasm and enlargement of the smooth muscle cells within the airway walls causing bronchospasm and wheezing.

The low oxygen in COPD causes constriction of small pulmonary arteries and thus increased pulmonary blood vessel resistance. This leads to pulmonary hypertension, or high blood pressure, in the pulmonary arterial system. This system conducts blood from the right side of the heart into the lungs, blood coming from the body low in oxygen and high in carbon dioxide. The right side of the heart normally has a very thin wall compared to the left side, but as pulmonary hypertension worsens, the muscle of the right side of the heart thickens in response to try to keep blood flowing into the lungs. Over time patients with pulmonary hypertension develop edema or swelling in their extremities and worsening of their shortness of breath. It also causes the patient to be very easily fatigued and lightheaded, and even cause chest pain and palpitations. The most ominous symptom is syncope, or fainting. It signifies that the right side of the heart cannot increase heart work load to meet the demands of even the simplest physical activity.

I first met Maddy when she was 72 years old with only traces of her once-beautiful blonde hair left amidst the gray, which she wore cut just below her ears. Her once attractive figure was long gone, her chest hyperexpanded in order to try to meet the oxygen needs of her body, so common in patients with COPD. Her skin was prematurely aged like most longtime smokers, had many blemishes or blotches of pigmentation with an ashen cast. She also had distention of her abdomen. Patients with COPD invariably swallow a lot of air trying to overcome their shortness of breath; it is this swallowed air that gives them the look of obesity. At this point in her life, Maddy had been smoking for over forty years, and it had certainly taken its toll on her.

She came to me initially as her previous doctor had left town, and a friend had recommended me. Maddy told me she had briefly passed out trying to climb their basement stairs, and this had scared Ralph considerably. She said she had had many episodes of lightheadedness before, but this was the first time she actually lost consciousness. In reviewing the records from her previous doctor, I saw that he had done quite a good job treating her COPD with bronchodilators and a combination medication with a twelve-hour bronchodilator plus a corticosteroid. For acute shortness of breath Maddy used a nebulizer. "Nebula" is the Latin word for cloud. The nebulizer machine makes a fog or cloud of medication for the patient to inhale. Since the smaller a particle is the deeper it gets into the lungs, the nebulizer is much more effective for these patients than a hand-held inhaler.

Maddy already had pulmonary hypertension with swelling of her legs and was on medication for this, including a digitalis preparation, a diuretic, and a vasodilator. However, her symptoms of shortness of breath and fluid retention were getting worse. I scheduled her for an echocardiogram, an ultrasound of the heart, to see how well her heart was pumping as well as how badly thickened the wall of the right side of her heart had become. Since her previous doctor had not started her on home oxygen, I also ordered the tests which would qualify her for Medicare coverage for this. I had her scheduled back a week later to review the test results.

When I received her results and even before Maddy came back, I contacted the cardiologist to discuss Maddy's case. He recommended that we have Maddy try a new medication, one initially investigated for pulmonary hypertension, yet later FDA-approved for one of its side effects. Though its effect on pulmonary hypertension was modest, it might help her by lowering the pulmonary pressures somewhat so she would be less short of breath, have less swelling, and be able to move about more easily. He advised she take a tablet twice a day at the lowest available dose. When Maddy return my office, I explained her tests showed rather severe pulmonary hypertension and told her what the cardiologist had recommended. She agreed to try the medication, and quite surprisingly, we were able to get her insurance company to agree to cover it.

For the next four months, the last four months of her life, she took one of those tablets twice daily every day. The medication gave her a significant decrease in swelling and shortness of breath. She could also walk well enough now to attend church for the first time in several years. After four months on her new medication, Maddy died in her sleep from a massive stroke, fortunately without suffering the suffocation so common in end-stage COPD.

Each time I saw Maddy after she began the new mediation, she always joked about it, telling Ralph that he ought to try it since it gave her "so much pep". She teased him saying he was always "down", and this would help to get him "up". She often laughed about her medicine, saying, "What a hoot!" As she knew its approved FDA indication, she always enjoyed joking with us and Ralph about her medicine. The new medication Maddy found so humorous was sildenafil, now FDA approved for pulmonary hypertension under the name Revatio, its name back then - Viagra.

Sacroiliitis

With the advent now of controversial state-run socialized medicine, many so-called experts fear that there are not enough primary care doctors available now or in the near future to handle the presumed increased workload expected to come with socialized medicine. Of course, many of these patients have been treated all along by those same primary care physicians, often at reduced rates or no charge at all, but the experts don't take this into account. Now several states are considering changing their laws to allow physician assistants or nurse practitioners to practice with no physician oversight.

As much as state-run socialized medicine is a sea-change for my profession, even more so would be the expansion of the scope of practice for physician assistants and nurse practitioners. Family physicians must train for approximately 21,000 hours to progress through medical school and residency to board certification. Currently nurse practitioners train only 3,500 to 6,000 hours. Moreover, some nurse practitioner schools are entirely online, thus providing no direct patient contact or supervision by more experienced faculty.

Some "experts" actually praise this difference in training and insist that nurse practitioners are more patient-centered than family physicians. This is an insult to those of us who have been in family medicine for decades. Moreover, I personally have found that this difference in training can lead to some rather poor patient outcomes, due to the relatively superficial training of the nurse practitioner compared to that of the family doctor. As one of my professors in neurology once told me, family medicine is the most demanding of all specialties, as the family doctor must know such a broad spectrum of medical information as well as understand one's own limitations and when to make a proper and timely referral to a more limited specialist. Development of this quality of professional judgment and understanding just does not happen in only 3,500 hours of training. Unfortunately, even with 21,000 hours of training, some family doctors fail to acquire such critical judgment. A few years ago, I met a patient named Phoebe, whose experience highlights this issue.

When I first met Phoebe, she was ninety-six years old and unable to stand up straight. I saw her as she was walking to the exam room, bent over at the waist and clutching a cane in each hand due to severe low back pain. My nurse assisted her onto the examining table, and I began visiting with Phoebe about the history of her problem. For the past two years she had been seeing a local nurse practitioner, who worked under a physician that was never present when the nurse practitioner was seeing patients. Phoebe had told this nurse practitioner of the low back pain she had had for several months, and how it seemed to radiate to her right hip and even at times into her right thigh. It was worse with certain activities such as having to stand in line at the local grocery store, and relieved by lying down on her left side. Even prolonged sitting was painful for her, except in her recliner chair.

Without examining the sensory sensation in Phoebe's legs and feet, nor the strength of her various leg muscles, the nurse practitioner ordered an MRI of the lumbar spine, a procedure costing over $3,000. Naturally, given Phoebe's age, the MRI showed she had extensive disc degeneration and arthritic osteophyte ("spur") formation within her spine at multiple levels. The nurse practitioner then referred Phoebe for a series of three epidural cortisone shots to be administered by the local radiologist. Unfortunately, she received little relief from these injections, and her pain continued unabated. The nurse practitioner then wrote her a prescription for an anti-inflammatory, a medication Phoebe had already tried that had failed to relieve her pain. She then had to live with the pain for several more months until her daughter, herself over sixty years old, came to visit. Her daughter told Phoebe she really needed to see a family doctor. Phoebe agreed but had been unable to do so as she could no longer drive, and she just didn't want to "bother" others by asking them to help her with transportation. It was this daughter who had brought Phoebe to my office that day.

After listening to Phoebe's story, I examined her in detail. She had normal sensation throughout both legs and feet. Although she had muscle atrophy and weakness from aging, this was symmetric in both legs. She specifically had no sign of nerve root compression, or radiculopathy, with electric shock-like pain down her legs or burning sensations, called paraesthesias, in any nerve distribution in her legs. It was then obvious that all of the abnormalities seen on the MRI of the lower back were all related to her advanced age but not due to nerve root impingement. There had to be another cause for her pain.

I asked Phoebe to try to localize her pain, as much as she possibly could, so I would get a better understanding of how and why she was hurting. She then reached behind and put her hand over the right side of her pelvis, telling me that the pain started there and ran down into her right hip. I then examined her pelvis and found she had marked irregularity and exquisite tenderness of the right sacroiliac joint.

Sacroiliitis is the inflammation of one of the joints between the sacrum and the iliac bones. The sacrum is the bottom part of the spine, and the iliac bones are the large pelvic bones which form a joint on each side with the sacrum. Sacroiliitis can cause pain in the buttock, lower back, and occasionally, as was the case with Phoebe, even pain down one or both legs. It is aggravated by prolonged standing or stair climbing. It can also be brought about by carrying more weight on one leg than another, especially if there is a difference in leg length. A sudden impact can also stress a sacroiliac joint as can simple osteo- or wear and tear-arthritis. Plain x-rays of the pelvis will often show signs of sacroiliitis and can be highly diagnostic. However, as was the case with Phoebe, a simple examination is often all that is necessary. Treatment for this disorder can involve physical therapy with range of motion exercises and stretching to maintain flexibility, a corticosteroid injection to the joint, destruction of the nerve causing the pain, implanting an electrical stimulator, or, as a last resort, surgical joint fusion to stop the pain.

In Phoebe's case her symptoms could be readily elicited with direct pressure on the right SI joint or by indirect stress. These maneuvers confirmed her diagnosis. I then prepared a combination injection of a corticosteroid with a local anesthetic. These two medications would be completely mixed in the syringe. If the local anaesthetic stopped her pain, we would then know the cortisone was in the right place. I prepped her skin and injected Phoebe's right sacroiliac joint. Within moments the local anesthetic would begin working. As Phoebe sat up from the injection, she was shocked to find that the pain, from which she had been suffering for over two years, was completely gone. Phoebe was able to step down off the exam table by herself. She was now able to stand straight up for the first time in weeks, and she walked out of the room without using either of her two canes.

Later that month, Phoebe called to thank me for having taken the time to investigate her problem and for having provided her with such inexpensive, dramatic, and long-lasting relief. Nine months later I learned that Phoebe had passed away. She apparently had died from a sudden myocardial infarction, or heart attack, during her sleep. At least I had been able to help this ninety-six year old lady enjoy nine months free of pain from sacroiliitis, something that the nurse practitioner had failed to do for two years.

Scoliosis

I first saw Abby Stevens five years ago when her mother brought her in for a routine physical. The family was about to begin taking in foster children, and the state required each of the family members to have a physical examination. Abby was a pretty, lean, and athletic girl with long straight sandy brown hair and pale blue eyes ringed in a darker blue. She was a generally healthy 11 year-old girl, an excellent student, and an athlete participating in several sports including basketball and volleyball. In reviewing Abby's history I found that she had had no significant medical problems, surgeries, or allergies. I thought her physical examination would be rather routine. It was not.

As I began examining Abby, I found no abnormalities with her eyes, ears, nose, or throat. However, just prior to listening to her chest and heart, I ran my hand down her back to see if it was straight. Sadly, it was anything but. Though the remainder of her examination appeared normal, my examination of her back showed a side-to-side S-shaped curvature of her spine curving to the right in the chest, or thoracic, area and to the left in the lower, or lumbar, area. This S-shaped curvature of her spine was quite pronounced and was to have a major impact on her life over the next year.

Scoliosis is the medical term for the lateral side-to-side curvature of the spine affecting Abby. It can be caused by a variety of neurologic and musculoskeletal disorders, but in the vast majority of cases, such as hers, there are no underlying causes found, so-called idiopathic scoliosis with no known cause. This disorder can be found in 2% to 4% of children in this country between the ages of ten and sixteen. To be diagnosed as scoliosis the curvature of the spine has to be greater than 10° as measured on spine x-rays, taken with the patient standing, and accompanied by rotation of the vertebral bodies. Of those diagnosed with scoliosis only 10% have any progression of their curvature requiring medical treatment. With very slight curvature boys and girls are equally affected, but with curvature greater than 30° girls outnumber boys ten to one. Also, scoliosis tends to progress more often in girls, so it is more common for them to need treatment than the boys. Yet I have had adult male patients who had to undergo surgery for scoliosis when the curvature became so bad that it interfered with heart and lung function.

In the 1970s school programs for scoliosis screening became quite popular. However, at the present time this has fallen out of favor. It seems too many children were being referred for specialist evaluation for what were really insignificant curvatures. Since 1990 there has been a marked decrease in such screening programs. Children are screened for scoliosis with a forward bending test called the Adams test. The child bends down at the waist, arms extended out together reaching toward the toes, then slowly coming back to an upright position. The screener looks for an abnormal prominence of the ribs and/or shoulder blade on one side of the back compared to the other. This test is still recommended by orthopedic specialists, but is to be performed by a physician to reduce the rate of unnecessary referrals.

When scoliosis has been newly diagnosed, the first concern is detection of any underlying clause, and the second is determining whether or not the curvature is likely to progress. The estimated future growth potential and the curvature at the time of diagnosis are both critical to predicting risk of progression. Again, girls have a risk of progression ten times higher than that of boys. The greater the growth potential and the larger the degree of curvature at initial diagnosis, the greater the likelihood of progression of the scoliotic curvature.

The child's growth potential is assessed by defining their level of puberty, called Tanner staging, and estimating the maturation of the iliac crest, the rim of the pelvic bone from front to back, called the Risser grade. The time just after the beginning of the adolescent growth spurt is usually the time of maximum progression of scoliotic curvatures. Evaluation of these various factors allows the physician to estimate the risk of curvature progression and is critical in timing an appropriate referral to the orthopedic specialist for definitive treatment.

The treatment for scoliosis includes bracing and, ultimately, surgery, as mentioned above. The use of a back brace can prevent significant progression of the curvature but will not correct that which has already developed. The older Milwaukee brace, with a support at the back of the head and under the chin, is still sometimes needed, but most cases can now be treated with an underarm brace worn under the clothing.

With this less embarrassing brace, children are much more likely to wear it day and night as required. Yet even with bracing about a fourth of the affected children will still have progression of their curvature and require surgery. In general it is believed that surgery should be performed for curvatures greater than 40° to 45° especially if the child is continuing to grow. It is best, if possible, to postpone surgery until the skeleton has stop growing, but if the curvature progresses quickly and at a young age, the orthopedic surgeon will implant rods whose length can be adjusted as the child continues to grow.

In Abby's case she had a 33° and 34° of curvature in the lumbar and thoracic areas, respectively, on her initial x-ray. She was just beginning her pubertal growth spurt, and of course, she was a girl. In her case, unfortunately, the curvatures in her chest and lower back progressed dramatically within eight months of her initial diagnosis, and her Risser grade showed she still had significant growing left to do. She was referred to a scoliosis specialist at the nearby university medical center where she underwent surgery to insert rods to straighten her back and stop the progression of curvature. Although this was quite a bit for an 11½-year-old girl to deal with, she accepted it well, and she was quite pleased to find that she had gained 3" in height from the operation.

Abby is now a happy, attractive 16 year-old with a steady boyfriend, the last I heard. I saw them enjoying a lunch together at a local restaurant, and I noticed how her posture was much better than his! She has adjusted well to the rigidity of her spine since her surgery, and she has been saved from severe deformity and the heart and lung problems that can occur with uncorrected advanced scoliosis.

It still surprises me, though, that in spite of her many previous well-child and sports physical examinations, her scoliosis had never been noted until I saw her that day for a foster care physical with an already advanced 33° curvature in her back. Maybe there is yet a role for better screening programs and earlier detection.

Subacute Combined Degenerative Neuropathy

"May you live in 'interesting' times," says an old Chinese curse, and Sue certainly lived an "interesting" life. Born on a rural farm, she was inflicted with verbal, physical, and sexual abuse as a child. Looking through the loving eyes of a child, the parent is seen as the one who knows what is best for you. Thus, when abused by that parent, you feel this was a just "punishment", implying that you somehow deserve it because you are "bad", completely undermining any sense of self-worth you might have. In addition, Sue was given excessive numbers of chores at an excessively young age. In her family your value as a person was based solely on what she did, rather than simply being the child that she was.

Sue left home at age seventeen, as soon as she graduated from high school and could get out of that home. A tall, attractive blond with a near-ideal figure, she was able to get a job right away working as a teller in a bank and attending college in the evenings, paying her own way through. After two years she married her first husband, her high school sweetheart, the first person who had ever been kind to her. Sadly, this man proved to be abusive like her father. She divorced him and later that marriage was annulled. Finally, Sue met a good man, who married her for who she was instead of what she looked like. He helped Sue both financially and emotionally, and she completed her masters degree in English. Along the way they had a daughter, and right afterward Sue had to undergo consecutive surgeries for bilateral carpal tunnel syndrome, the compression of the median nerve at the wrist causing numbness and tingling in the hands. At the same time Sue had to begin her student teaching. Since she had always been driven to work hard, having so much "on her plate" at one time did not stop her.

Sue still felt at that point that she had value only for what she did rather than for just being who she was. Finally Sue had "made it", now having completed her master's degree and beginning to teach at the high school level.

Unfortunately, Sue had been a vegetarian on and off for years without taking supplemental vitamin B12. Sue began having symptoms of B12 deficiency, initially with numbness and tingling in her hands, which she attributed to recurrence of carpal tunnel syndrome. She chose to ignore it. She was too busy with her life to have any time to "be sick" or pay attention to herself. Soon the numbness and tingling, known as paresthesias, began in her feet and legs as well. Now she was dropping things, had an abnormal gait, and was losing excessive weight.

Sue was becoming short-tempered with extreme fatigue. She would lay down for a nap after work and not wake up until midnight. Still she felt she could not let up with her constantly busy schedule. When she started having spasms and cramps in her legs, it became so bad that a muscle spasm in her leg caused her to miss the brake and wreck her car. Finally, after three years with these symptoms, Sue collapsed while working on her computer at home. Her husband took her to the emergency room of the local hospital, where she was found to have a very low B12 level in her blood. Inexplicably, she was sent home, nearly paralyzed by the neuropathy, and having severe pain with hyperesthesia. This last refers to extreme reaction to the slightest stimulus; it felt as if her skin had first been peeled off when she would feel the brushing of clothing against her leg or a light touch on her arm. The pain was extreme.

At that time my wife and I were visiting our children and grandchildren out of state. Desperate, Sue's husband contacted our local hospital and was finally able to reach me in Michigan. He explained to me what was happening to Sue and that her B12 level had been extremely low.

Since Sue had never confided in me that she had been experiencing these symptoms, progressively worsening for three years, I was completely surprised to learn all this. I advised him to take Sue immediately to the medical center in the nearby large city. I advised him I would call to arrange for a trusted neurologist to see Sue there at once.

When she arrived, she underwent multiple tests to rule out other causes of her condition. These led the neurologist very quickly to diagnose Sue with subacute combined degenerative neuropathy, the neuropathy of prolonged vitamin B12 deficiency.

Subacute combined degenerative neuropathy, abbreviated SCD, produces neurologic symptoms including memory impairment, poor attention span, changes in mood, and even trouble with vision. It also causes the pins-and-needles sensation and muscle spasms and tics such as Sue had been experiencing. These symptoms progress symmetrically in a distal to proximal fashion, that is to say, from toes to thigh, leading to unsteady gait, poor coordination, and the loss of position sense. Sue could not close her eyes and bring her index finger to her nose. All of these neurologic findings are complemented with extreme pain.

At the medical center Sue had an MRI of spine which demonstrated an abnormally white signal in the posterior columns of the spinal cord. This signified demyelinization of these nerve tracks. The myelin around the nerves is like the insulation on a wire. Once this is removed, the neural signals are completely scrambled, leading to the symptoms which Sue had been experiencing.

Unfortunately, any significant delay in diagnosis or treatment leads to little or no improvement, even with complete B12 replacement. Sue had ignored these symptoms for three years until they became so severe she could ignore them no longer. Sue had to face the fact that because of this delay, she now had irreversible injury to the spinal cord and nerves with no prospect for improvement. Her condition was now permanent.

Initially Sue was treated with physical therapy, itself quite painful. She then had to go through the process of chronic pain management. This always begins with milder measures, such as a TENS unit and anti-inflammatory medications, both of which proved to be completely ineffective for her. She was tried on several medications normally used for neuropathy, and either they were not helpful or their side effects were intolerable.

We finally tried Cymbalta which did help. In addition, I had to titrate, or gradually adjust upward, the dosage of a sustained-action narcotic medication to get Sue's pain under control. She would also take another short-acting narcotic medication for "breakthrough" pain. On those days when the pain was worse, such as with weather changes, Sue dreads even getting out of bed, but at least the breakthrough pain medication makes it tolerable on those bad days. Lastly, I had to add another medication to control muscle spasms and tics.

It took almost eight years to get Sue's medicine adjusted so that she could function even somewhat normally again. The medications cause constipation, but she has been able to control this with diet and the stool softeners. On her present regimen Sue can walk fairly well with a cane, go up and down stairs on her buttocks, and scoot along the floor to do dusting and other light housework. She has now come to the understanding that she has value as a human being, regardless of what she can do or accomplish.

Sue stays quite active, visiting with others having problems as bad, if not worse, than her own. She has spent hours with the dying, comforting the spouse, and helping them to face what they are enduring. Through helping others she has found great value even in her life of disability. Sue has overcome trials that would have crushed a lesser person. She knows now that her life has value simply because she is living it.

Success

Although racial prejudice is nearly universally condemned in American society now, it still exists but in a more subtle form. Other types of prejudice, often much more open, are now much more common and even "acceptable", particularly in urban coastal states. One such prejudice is based on regional origin. Terms such as "hayseed", "hick", or even "dirt-ball" are often used toward those from the rural south or central states. Those in urban areas of the East or West coast tend to look down on those from what they like to refer to as "fly-over country".

A similar prejudice is often seen toward one's lack of formal education. Those without a college degree or more especially, a high school diploma, are frequently looked down upon by those who have themselves completed their university education (and thus should know better). Yet some with advanced degrees can still confuse ignorance with lack of intelligence. Such people also frequently mistake their knowledge for the wisdom they so often lack.

Finally, there is a third open prejudice against those with large families. Such bigoted people consider children to be a burden rather than a blessing. They will often make hurtful, derogatory comments to parents of such families, comments often far worse than those harboring racial prejudice would ever make face-to-face to someone of another race.

Henry and Mae Jackson had been subject to all three of these prejudices, yet theirs was one of the most wonderful families I have ever met.

I first met the Jacksons when Mae was hospitalized at the university medical center for diabetes, now needing insulin. They had driven up to the medical center in Henry's old pickup truck, Mae wearing a simple green house dress, her hair braided behind her, while Henry wore an old straw hat, worn jeans, work-beaten cowboy boots, and a faded western shirt, the kind with the fake pearl snaps. They looked like any poor rural couple coming out of the hills of eastern Kentucky.

As an intern, I did Mae's initial evaluation. After me came the resident, and it was obvious to all three of us that he held some, if not all, of the prejudices mentioned above. While the resident was interviewing and examining Mae, I asked Henry if he would like some coffee, since it was late. He agreed, and I showed him the way to the hospital cafeteria, where we shared a few cups of coffee while Henry shared with me the rest of their story.

Henry had dropped out of high school when he was just sixteen years old. He had taken a job working for "old man Miller" at his gas station in the small rural Kentucky town near his family's farm. His father had died from black lung disease that year, and Henry felt he needed to work to help support his mother and sister. In two years' working at the gas station Henry saved every extra penny, enough so he felt he could marry Mae, his childhood sweetheart, who had just graduated from high school. They moved in with his family while he continued working at the gas station. Mae did all she could to keep their expenses down, living as simply as possible to help Henry save for their future.

By the time they were twenty years old, Henry and Mae had two children and a few thousand dollars saved. That year Mr. Miller had his second heart attack and finally decided to retire. Henry talked it over with Mae, and since Henry was good at running the gas station, they decided to use their savings to buy it.

Continuing to keep expenses to a minimum, after another two years and another child, they had saved enough for Henry to buy a used grader with a scoop on the back. Mae was not sure about this, wondering why Henry wanted to spend their savings for this piece of heavy equipment. However, through selling him diesel fuel for the last several years, Henry had become good friends with the man who had the road contract with the county - grading the unpaved roads in the summer, and plowing the snow off the paved ones in the winter.

He told Henry he was not going to renew his contract with the county. Henry bid the same amount his predecessor was paid, and his bid was accepted. With his grader, Henry did the work for the county in the evenings after working at the gas station during the day. Now with two businesses bringing in income, Henry and Mae were able to save even more.

Another three years went by as Henry and Mae had their third and fourth children and, still living on as little as possible, had again saved several thousand dollars. Henry's mother had passed away shortly after the birth of their fourth child, leaving Henry the family farm. Like many of the rural farms in eastern Kentucky, much of the land was too vertical to be tillable. Henry knew that beneath the soil on their mountain was a vast amount of high-quality coal, but he also knew he could not legally "mine" it.

But Henry discovered another way, a way that would keep him from getting into trouble about strip mining while fulfilling a federal contract!

The federal government had purchased a "holler" on the edge of town where a low-income housing project would be built. For this project, the government needed fill dirt and lots of it. Henry was more than willing to oblige, and, once again submitting the low bid, he got the job.

With their savings Henry now bought another piece of used equipment, a large diesel dump truck. With this and his grader/scoop he began supplying the fill dirt for the new project, dirt which Henry carefully removed off the top of his coal each evening, after the gas station closed and the road grading was done. By the time Henry had fulfilled his federal contract to supply the fill dirt, most of the coal on their land was uncovered. Now Henry became a coal operator.

Henry and Mae were in their late forties when they had their sixth and seventh children. Their two eldest were attending college, and three more were in high school. They owned a gas station, a coal mine, and a road grading business. While Mae was in the hospital, I was able to meet the entire family, including all seven of the children.

One of the older children revealed to me that Henry and Mae had over $2 million in net worth. One would never have guessed it from their simple, humble ways and appearance. Though some of my fellow physicians at the medical center looked down on Henry and Mae due to their lack of formal education, few of those doctors, though blessed with good education and great opportunities, would accomplish as much and Henry and Mae, who had started out with no economic or educational advantages.

Mae was only at the medical center for four days until her diabetes was under good control - now with insulin, and Henry could take her home. After she was discharged, I thought that was the last I would hear from them, but three years later Henry called me. Their eldest had been accepted to a prestigious medical school, and Henry and Mae couldn't have been prouder. Mae had lost weight, and her diabetes was under very good control, now without insulin. Henry was still in good health and working every day. He had grown up in rural eastern Kentucky, never finished high school, married while still a teenager, raised seven children, and now was paying his son's way through medical school. The Henry and Mae Jackson family was a success.

Thunderstorm

It was a brisk, cool spring morning as I left to go to the hospital for rounds that day. Though the morning sky was a bright blue, there was an ominous line of dark clouds off to the west. As I got into my car to drive to the hospital, I could smell the coming rain. At the hospital I had two patients, a young Amish woman and her newborn baby delivered the evening before. That morning I would discharge both of them. Everything having gone well through the night, so there was no reason for them to have to stay longer.

I explained the plan for follow-up care to her and her husband, dictated her discharge summary, wrote her prescriptions, and did the same for the infant. Lastly, I called my office to arrange time for a house call the next day to check on her and the baby. Once again, as I left the hospital to walk over to my office, I could smell the coming rain.

We had a fairly light schedule in the office that morning, and as it turned out, this was a blessing. About ten o'clock that morning the rain began, heralded by an intense show of lightning and thunder. Shortly after the rain became heavy we got a call from the emergency room.

I was informed that a patient of mine, an old German farmer named John Williams, had been struck by lightning while working at his farm and was being brought by ambulance to the emergency room. They would arrive within minutes. I quickly finished with the patient I was seeing and hurried to the emergency room to await the arrival of the ambulance.

John Williams had been a very active, hard-working farmer all of his adult life. John and his wife raised four children, but only one was interested in farming. The youngest son, John Jr., had attended Michigan State University where he obtained his degree in agriculture with a minor in business administration.

After graduation he was immediately able to help his father with the family farm, particularly with financial asset management. John was rather proud of John Jr., though being an old-school German farmer, he would never tell his son that. By age sixty-five, however, John had decided it was time to step aside and allow his son gradually to assume management of the farm. Having always been an avid hunter and fisherman, John enjoyed these avocations while still helping out at times and advising John Jr. about agricultural matters. John had always been a lean fellow, but he had been putting on weight the last few years of his semi-retirement as he was quite a bit less active physically.

The ambulance arrived shortly after I did, and the crew brought John in on a hard board with a splint on his right arm. As I was beginning a systematic evaluation of John, the EMTs informed me that John had been helping his son hurry to finish planting a field before the rain broke. They finished their work just as the storm began. John was heading back along the edge of the field beside their pole fence when the tractor he was riding was struck by lightning. He was thrown at least fifteen feet in the air and had come down straddling the pole fence. He was clearly in a lot of pain.

The EMTs wheeled John into the trauma room and raised him up still on the board, placing him on the gurney. John was barely conscious. In Advanced Trauma Life Support (ATLS) one is taught a specific sequence in evaluating the trauma victim. As in Advanced Cardiac Life Support (ACLS), the first step is to make sure the patient has a good airway and is breathing. Circulation, heart function, and evidence of significant bleeding are next quickly assessed. Then a thorough evaluation of the body ensues, all done in a quick, systematic manner following well-established protocols so that the trauma team does not overlook any significant injury.

One obvious injury John had was to his heart. Though John was not actually directly struck by the lightning bolt, the electricity around his body had triggered multiple irregular beats which we noted as soon as we had him attached to the electronic monitor. As we started two large bore IVs to maintain blood pressure and circulation, we gave him lidocaine through one of them. This, fortunately, rapidly resolved the ectopy, or abnormal heartbeats.

We noted John's right upper arm was angulated bizarrely with a large fracture hematoma, a collection of blood under the skin from a blood vessel ruptured with the fracture. We also found his right leg was abnormally rotated inward, his right toes pointing at his left heel. Then, as we cut away his clothing, we saw he had blood coming from the penis. Fortunately, as we completed his total body evaluation, we found no more major injuries.

We obtained x-rays of John's head, chest, right arm, right leg, and pelvis. These demonstrated a simple displaced fracture of the right upper arm, a comminuted (multiple pieces) fracture of the right hip, and several displaced fractures of the pelvis. When the nurse attempted to insert a urinary catheter, she said it felt like the catheter would not go into the bladder, and all she could get was blood. I immediately had her stop her efforts, changed gloves, and did a careful rectal exam. Though there was no blood in his rectum, I could not feel John's prostate. He had come down so hard on the pole fence that the blow to his pelvis not only shattered bone but also severed his urethra at its origin on the urinary bladder. The urethra is the tube carrying urine from the bladder to the outside. This injury caused the so-called "high-riding" prostate on exam.

As John's blood pressure and pulse were stabilized and his injuries immobilized, I called the referral hospital in Kalamazoo and spoke with their urologist as well as their orthopedist on-call. Both specialists would be standing by, awaiting John's arrival by helicopter. As I later learned, they decided to work together. The urologist reattached John's urethra to his bladder while the orthopedist repaired John's multiple fractures, all during a single episode of general anesthesia. When the two specialists finally finished working on John, he was transferred from the operating room to the hospital's surgical intensive care unit, where he spent the next few weeks. After that, he was transferred to a rehab facility to complete his recovery.

Given the extent of John's injuries, I was not surprised that was a few months later, well into the summer, before I saw him again. He came to my office to thank me for what we had done that fateful day in the emergency room. The injuries had left John with a slight limp in his gait, but he told me that he no longer had any pain. He was able to urinate normally and was once again helping out around the farm.

His son, John Jr., had been reluctant to let his father do very much at first, but he finally realized that letting his father do what he could was important to his recovery, both physically and mentally. John had returned to semi-retired farming again, but as he put it, "Now I have much greater respect for thunderstorms."

Where's Mama?

"Doctor, I've been feeling very tired. I haven't had much appetite, yet I have been gaining weight. I don't understand how, since I eat only a few bites before I feel full. My bathroom scales don't show I've gained much, but most of my dresses don't fit anymore around the middle. This has been going on for several months, but I put off seeing the doctor because of Oliver, my husband, who has Alzheimer's disease. Today a long-time friend is staying with him while I came here. What made me finally decide to come was that for the last few weeks I have been short of breath, and this week I suddenly had arthritis pains in my hips, knees, and feet. I guess I should just expect things like that at my age."

These were the words of Geneva Phillips, whom I was seeing for the first time. Each an only-child, Geneva and Oliver had married when she was twenty-five and he thirty. He ran the "mom-and-pop" hardware store started by his father; she was an elementary school teacher. They had met at church, fallen in love, and married.

Unfortunately, as much as Geneva loved children, they were never able to have any of their own. Yet theirs was a happy life together. She had retired from teaching due to her age. Oliver had to close the hardware store due to competition from major chain stores and problems managing the store; he was in the first stages of

Alzheimer's disease. It was much worse when I saw Geneva. Oliver's previous doctor recommended a nursing home for him, but she adamantly refused. Both of Oliver's parents had died in a nursing home, and Oliver had made her promise never to put him in one. Though she had never been able to have her own children, Geneva had taken care of thousands of children as a teacher over the years. Now she had just one, the child-like Oliver, who depended on her for everything.

It was a pleasure talking with Geneva, a very proper lady-like woman seventy-five years of age. She wore her hair in a tight bun on the back of her head, wire-rimmed bifocal glasses, and a modest floral house dress. As I listened to her, I couldn't help thinking to myself how many patients claim they hardly ate a thing yet kept gaining weight. Sadly, this was not the case with her. The overall impression that she gave was of someone feeling very bad, yet her symptoms were vague and nonspecific.

On examination I found she had decreased breath sounds over the base of the right lung as compared to the left. Her dresses were no longer fitting well because her abdomen was distended with fluid. Given these findings, it was obvious that additional testing would be necessary. We scheduled her for blood tests and CAT scans of her chest, abdomen, and pelvis. I would see her back in three days to review the results with her. She agreed to have the tests done as she felt confident her friend would agree to stay with Oliver at the time of her testing and for her return visit. Geneva then very courteously but firmly refused any hospitalization; she simply would not leave Oliver at a nursing home, nor did she wish to leave him for more than a few hours. She told me Oliver was the only man she'd ever loved, a man with whom she had spent most of her life, and now her life was centered around caring for him. I nodded and let her know that I understood how she felt and would try to respect that.

Unfortunately, the CAT scans showed a large mass where her right ovary would have been, free fluid throughout the abdomen and around her right lung, with hundreds of small tumors in her liver, in the abdominal fat, and on the peritoneum, the membrane lining the abdominal cavity. Geneva had end-stage ovarian cancer.

Cancer of the ovary is the sixth most common cancer in women. Far more important than the number of cases is that the vast majority of women with these cancers initially present with advanced disease as did Geneva. Their overall survival is thus much worse than with other types of cancer.

There is no clear causative factor for ovarian cancers, but population-based data show that those with the fewest menstrual cycles throughout life have the fewest ovarian cancers. Such women may have had multiple pregnancies and nursed all their babies, or may have started late and ended early. Conversely, those like Geneva, who had never been pregnant or used birth-control pills, had the highest number of menstrual cycles in their lifetime and were thus at greatest risk. Sadly, there are no specific symptoms of ovarian cancer. There can be abdominal bloating, discomfort, loss of appetite, fatigue, and with advanced disease, even a cancer-induced arthritis.

The spread of ovarian cancer within the abdomen produces free abdominal fluid, known as ascites, as Geneva had. There are many types of ovarian cancers. Some respond well to chemotherapy while others respond poorly, if at all. Unfortunately, there is no evidence that any screening, including tumor markers such as CA-125 by blood testing or even periodic ultrasound can detect early stage ovarian cancer.

Upon her return I explained to Geneva the findings of her CAT scans and blood tests. We discussed her concerns about Oliver, along with my concerns about getting a definite tissue diagnosis. She gently reminded me that she would not agree to surgery or hospitalization. However, she agreed to let me remove some of the fluid from her abdomen to relieve her pressure symptoms and shortness of breath. The cells found in this fluid might also confirm her diagnosis.

With her consent I performed the paracentesis, the procedure for removing ascites fluid, there in the office. We were able to remove four liters of fluid, after which she felt much better. I sent the fluid to the laboratory for examination. The pathologist examined the cells in it, including doing some special staining of them, and confirmed this was an adenocarcinoma of the ovary, likely of the mucinous type, one of the poorest in responding to chemotherapy.

Upon her return three days later, I explained to Geneva the findings on the ascites fluid. She gently and graciously informed me that all she now needed from me was medication for her discomfort, should she require it. She would just go home and take care of Oliver. She wanted nothing further done.

I explained to her that if we did not take care of her, she would not be there to take care of Oliver. She patted me gently on the arm, saying, "I know, young man, but I know my duty and what I must do."

That was the last time I saw Geneva Phillips. The next I heard of her was from the local police. They called to tell me that a neighbor had found Oliver wandering in the street in his pajamas, asking, "Where's Mama? Where's Mama?"

The neighbor gently guided Oliver back home, explored the house, and found Geneva where she had died in her sleep. As Mr. and Mrs. Phillips had no living family, I called the county attorney right away. He arranged for a court-ordered guardian for Oliver, who was then admitted to a nursing home, where he spent his final days. Each time I saw him in the nursing home, he would always ask me, "Where's Mama?"

Oliver died within a year of Geneva. His death certificate said "Alzheimer's disease", but I think it was more from grief.

White Coat

I still remember the beginning of my third-year in medical school when we were finally allowed to wear a white coat. These were white jackets extending just below the waist, with large pockets for our papers, equipment, and clinical notebooks. This marked a turning point in our medical careers, for we were embarking on bedside patient care for the first time as doctors in training. There would be many more years ahead before we would be allowed to wear the full length long lab coats the attending physicians wore, but we were proud of having made it even to that milestone. Since I was a medical student decades ago, there has emerged a "White Coat Ceremony" at many medical schools to mark that transition.

Until the late 19th-century, doctors dressed in black formal attire to emphasize the seriousness of their work, even in the operating room. The number of blood stains on a doctor's coat indicated how successful he was and how many patients he was seeing.

Yet doctors were often seen as quacks and charlatans whose treatments were useless or worse. It wasn't until the germ theory of disease and concepts of asepsis were widely accepted that medicine started to become scientific.

Thanks to the work of such pioneers as Lister and Pasteur, it was shown beyond a doubt that antiseptic techniques could prevent bacterial contamination and thus disease.

By the late 1880s doctors began wearing white coats to demonstrate their avoidance of germs. The 1910 Flexner report led to the closure of hundreds of inferior medical institutions and the standardization of modern scientific medical education. By this time cleanliness and aseptic technique had become central to the practice of medicine.

During this past century the white coat remained the premier symbol of medical authority and respect and aided in establishing the doctor-patient relationship. Seeing someone on television wearing a long white coat, one reflexively assumes the wearer was a physician.

However, this image has also been felt to be so intimidating that psychiatrists and many pediatricians have abandoned them. These specialists seem to feel that not wearing the white coat reduces their patients' anxiety. They cite such phenomena as the so-called "white coat" hypertension which is blamed on the coat, but I have found that many patients have a higher blood pressure in my office than at home simply because they are seeing the doctor, regardless of what I am wearing.

Today there is still division about the use of the white coat in clinical settings. Supporters say that the white coat documents to the patient a physician's cleanliness and symbolizes their authority and trustworthiness. Those opposed see the white coat as a symbol that distances the doctor from the patient, putting the doctor on a pedestal above the patient.

The white coat is essentially universally worn at university medical centers, while doctors in smaller hospitals and in private practice are less likely to wear them. In 2009 the American Medical Association voted on a resolution recommending hospitals ban doctors' white coats, citing studies linking the coats to the spread of infection. Too often doctors have failed to wear a clean one each day, thus contributing to that problem.

Another study of the white coat showed that 56% of patients feel doctors should wear them while only 24% of doctors agreed. Older patients seemed to prefer the white coat more; they were much less likely to trust a doctor wearing scrubs instead. In my many years of practice there have been times when I've worn the white coat, and other times when I have chosen not to wear one.

Perhaps the most remarkable incident about wearing a white coat occurred for me in the summer of 2000 when our son, daughter-in-law, and grandchildren came from Michigan to visit us for a week. Just before their departure from home, our daughter-in-law noticed that one of the grandsons, Nicholas, just three years old, had nasal congestion and a periodic cough. He had also just begun running a low-grade fever. She brought along medication for Nicholas should he need it on the trip, and he seemed to be better with it. They arrived at our house that first evening very late, and the grandchildren were quickly put to bed for the night. Before putting Nicholas to bed, his mother again gave him some liquid acetaminophen for his fever and pain, and he seemed to do well after that through the rest of the night.

The next morning, though, his fever was back even higher. Now he was complaining that his ear hurt. His mother walked Nicholas the three blocks from our house to my office for me to check him. She told me about his congestion and cough and starting to have the low-grade fever the day before. She said he awoke that morning complaining of an earache.

When I asked him if his ear hurt, Nicholas nodded "yes" and pointed to his right ear. As I start examining him, Nicholas stared straight ahead at his mother, and I sensed he was somewhat frightened at seeing a doctor. I was, of course, wearing my white coat.

On examination I found his right ear was inflamed with the eardrum slightly bulging. He had a green mucus with the nasal congestion, slight redness in his throat, and a few enlarged tender lymph nodes on his neck under the right ear. The remainder of his examination was fairly normal.

I explained all this to his mother and wrote out prescriptions for Nicholas for antibiotic and an ear drop to help relieve his pain. Nicholas sat quietly while I was telling his mother all this. Before he left the office, I gave him a red lollipop as a reward for having behaved so well. I continued seeing other patients through that afternoon, but

I closed the office an hour early so Dianne and I could spend more time with our children and grandchildren.

When I got home, I asked Nicholas how he was doing. Since I had left my white coat in the office, Nicholas was seeing me in my regular clothes. He ran to me and said, "Grandpa, I went to see the doctor today!"

He then proceeded to tell me all about his visit to the doctor, that he had been given medicine for his sore ear, and that he even got a lollipop. When I reminded him it was a red one, he looked at me with surprise and said, "How did you know?"

I chuckled and reminded him that I was the doctor he had seen. Nicholas then became very serious, shook his head, and said slowly, "No, Grandpa, I saw the doctor today, not you." There was nothing I could say to convince him that I was the doctor he had seen. The white coat with its name tag and pockets full of instruments and papers had made that much of an impression upon him.

I don't know what the future will be for the medical white coat. It is still a major symbol for my profession, and I suspect it will remain so for a long time yet. If it is eventually abandoned, I am sure that the teaching hospitals will be the last to do so.

After my experience with Nicholas, I wonder if other doctors, working at such centers, go unrecognized by their grandchildren, too.

Yellow Jackets

If you have ever driven through eastern Kentucky, you may have noticed some unusual looking barns. They are very tall, moderately wide, and distinguished by characteristic rows of long, narrow, almost two-story high shutters, which can be opened on either side of the barn to let in air. These barns are essentially stacks of drying racks for tobacco. Inside the barns are several tiers spaced vertically about five feet apart, consisting of rows timbers spaced about three to four feet apart upon which tobacco stakes are placed for drying.

On these tobacco stakes, long straight sharpened sticks, the stems of freshly cut tobacco plants are impaled. The stakes are then placed across the timbers in each tier with the tobacco plants hanging upside down where they will be left to dry over the next many weeks. The tall narrow shutters on the sides of the barn are opened to allow breezes in and can be closed during heavy storms.

Once the plants are thoroughly dried, young men will climb the tiers of the barn and pass down the dried plants to another who will stack them on carts. The carts are then taken to the "stripping room" where the leaves will be stripped off the stalks, stacked and tied into bales, and the bales taken to be sold at the tobacco auction.

This story is about what once happened as a tobacco barn was being emptied.

Jake Patton was a thin, wiry nineteen year-old with a shock of pale blonde hair unruly as a haystack, intense blue eyes, a rather sparse scraggly blonde beard, and a warm smile that would melt butter. Even as a youngster he loved to climb, scrambling up trees with ease when he would go hunting with his father. It was thus no surprise that Jake would always be the first one to scurry up to the top of a tobacco barn and pass down the stakes with their dried tobacco plants to those more fearful of heights.

On this particular autumn day Jake and three of his friends had been hired to empty a neighbor's tobacco barn. They had nearly finished emptying the first side of the barn when Jake unfortunately struck a giant yellow jacket nest with the end of one of the tobacco stakes. His friends later told me that although Jake was a quick climber, they had never seen him move so fast as he did in the next few seconds.

Thousands of angry, aggressive wasps came pouring out of the nest, and Jake's head and upper body were quickly surrounded and covered by a huge swarm of yellow jackets. As fast as he was moving, he already had multiple stings before he reached the ground.

Jake hit the ground running, dashing out of the barn and then racing around the barnyard, screaming as loud as he could and flailing at the air with his arms. His companions ran out of the barn after him. It took them a long time to get Jake to stop running and try to calm down. Finally, two of them grabbed his arms and lead him quickly to their truck to bring him into town.

Jake kept yelling something which they initially couldn't understand, but finally one of them realized he was saying there was a yellow jacket in his ear. Unfortunately, it was unable to find its way out. The boys later told me they had never seen someone in such a panic, and no wonder.

The yellow jacket is a type of wasp identified by alternating black and yellow body segments or stripes and their small size. They are social wasps that live in a colony begun by a single queen. In the spring the queen begins by chewing plant fibers to create a paper-type nest and starts laying eggs. These hatch into sterile female worker wasps that expand the area of search for food. They also care for the queen and the immature wasps in the nest. A typical yellow jacket nest may contain between 500 to 15,000 cells and have several thousand worker wasps.

In parts of the South a mild winter followed by an early spring can lead to a colony of over 100,000 wasps. Each nest tends to reach its maximum size in early fall. The yellow jacket is known to be an aggressive defender of its colony. Unlike bees, each wasp can sting repeatedly. Most wasps will not sting unless provoked, but yellow jackets are an exception. They are very aggressive by nature, especially when foraging for the limited food left for them in the fall. Thus Jake had disturbed these nasty insects at perhaps the worst possible time.

I was just starting to see my last patient of the morning, scheduled for routine follow-up on blood pressure, when their pickup truck screeched to a stop in front of my office and all four young men ran inside, Jake still struggling to control his panic.

My nurse quickly got their story of what had happened and why Jake was dancing from one foot to the other and still yelling. She quickly escorted Jake into our treatment room and ran to get me. It was fortunate that Jake was not allergic to yellow jacket stings since he was peppered with dozens of them. He was shaking with fear with the wasp still crawling and scratching in his ear while its antennae scraped across his ear drum.

Back in the treatment room I enlisted the help of Jake's friends to hold him still on the table. With my otoscope, the instrument doctors use to look in the ear, I could see the hind segment of the wasp with its stinger just inside Jake's ear canal. Fortunately, I had learned a technique that helped greatly in this circumstance.

Reaching for a bottle of Marcaine, a local anesthetic, I quickly filled a syringe with it and used the syringe like a squirt gun to fill Jake's ear canal with Marcaine. At once the wasp stopped moving and was no longer able to hold its position in the ear canal. I then easily removed it from Jake's ear with forceps and crushed it. Jake became calm immediately. In addition, because he was covered with so many stings, I was concerned about the ultimate extent of

Jake's reaction to the total quantity of venom with which he had been injected. I gave Jake an injection of Benadryl, an antihistamine, to reduce his reaction to the venom and prescribed a short course of corticosteroid tablets as well as an antihistamine capsule. I advised Jake use ice to the stings to reduce the swelling and asked him to call me the next day to let me know how he was doing.

The next day Jake called my office to inform me that he was doing much better. He still had significant swelling, but it had not gotten any worse than when I had seen him in the office the day before. It was of interest to me that his panic that day had been so severe that he had little recollection of having been to my office.

That same day his companions returned to the barn, accompanied by the local exterminator, who had been called about the yellow jackets. Their nest was the size of a giant pizza pan, over two feet across, and contained tens of thousands of wasps. The exterminator was able to destroy the nest without further incident. Within another three days Jake's swelling was down, and he was back to his normal, cheerful self. Even today, in all my years of medical practice, Jake was the most frantic patient I have ever seen in my office.

Made in the USA
Lexington, KY
08 August 2016